Hormones

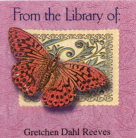

HORMONES

THE MESSENGERS OF LIFE

Lawrence Crapo

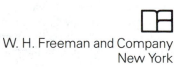
W. H. Freeman and Company
New York

This book was published originally as a volume of *The Portable Stanford*, a book series published by the Stanford Alumni Association, Stanford, California.

Library of Congress Cataloging in Publication Data

Crapo, Lawrence M., 1938-
   Hormones, messengers of life.

   Bibliography: p.
   Includes index.
   1. Hormones.   I. Title.
QP571.C73   1985   574.19′27   85-16065
ISBN 0-7167-1757-3
ISBN 0-7167-1753-0 (pbk.)

Printed in the United States of America
1 2 3 4 5 6 7 8 9 0 ML 4 3 2 1 0 8 9 8 7 6 5

This book is dedicated to
the memory of my friend Timothy Beckett,
whose untimely death from cancer in the prime of his life
deeply affected me. His remarkable courage,
exceptional talent as a physician, and innate good will
stand as a monument to human dignity.

CONTENTS

PREFACE

Several years ago in San Francisco I wandered into a Chinese restaurant for lunch with friends who were attending a scientific conference with me. I usually look forward to my fortune cookie—for that fleeting bit of wisdom that often makes one's day. On this occasion, however, I was rudely shifted out of my blissful postprandial torpor by a rather devastating message:

Stiff in opinion, always in the wrong!

This unsettling message is now posted on my office door to remind me and all who enter of the curious malady to which we in academic settings are particularly prone. With this in mind, I have tried hard in this book about hormones and other chemical messengers to keep the opinion guarded and the scientific facts at the forefront, even when it has occasionally resulted in slight hurdles for readers unfamiliar with my subject.

Many of the topics discussed in these pages are in the process of a rapid evolution created by the remarkable productivity of numerous investigative laboratories throughout the world. Consequently, some of the ideas expressed in this book will no doubt be rendered obsolete within the next five or ten years. Nevertheless, I have not backed away from these rapidly changing areas; they are intriguing to me, and my purpose in writing this book is to share with the general reader my own excitement about chemical messengers and how they influence our lives.

I have been helped immensely in this task by the incisive editing of Jane Bavelas and Miriam Miller. Whatever clarity has been achieved here is due in great part to their tenacious comments. I also wish to thank Laura Ackerman-Shaw and Pamela Manley for their help with the illustrations, and my wife Kathy for her support.

I suppose it is only just to acknowledge our dog Alyosha who spent endless nights with me, flopped on the rug, staring at me with his big inquiring Samoyed eyes, probably wondering if I really knew what I was doing, and certainly wondering when the next round of food was going to be served up.

Lawrence Crapo

Stanford University
August 1985

THE EVOLUTION OF
CHEMICAL MESSENGERS

■

Evolution behaves like a tinkerer, who, during eons upon eons, would slowly modify his work, unceasingly retouching it, cutting here, lengthening there, seizing the opportunities to adapt it progressively to its new use. . . . Evolution does not produce novelties from scratch. It works on what already exists, either transforming a system to give it new functions or combining several systems to produce a more elaborate one.
— François Jacob, "Evolution and Tinkering"

You could hardly imagine a more congested situation. Like an urban freeway on a late Friday afternoon, at any given moment our circulatory system is literally packed with chemical messengers—an endless tide of hormones passing through in search of receptors on distant target cells, where they will initiate a vital cascade of life-sustaining events inside of the cells. As though we were watching a sea of cars drive by on their way to some meaningful destination, we see the hormones in transit, holding things together and orchestrating the most complex network of physiology that nature has yet been able to devise: Thyroxine on its way from the thyroid gland in the neck to its own receptors inside of many different cells throughout the body to control the rate of metabolism; cortisol from the adrenal glands above the kidneys heading for its target cells; growth hormone making its way from the pituitary gland in the brain to the liver to stimulate production of growth factors; parathyroid hormone keeping your calcium in balance; insulin maintaining your serum glucose level right where it belongs; and on they go—a multitude of hormones, each pursuing its own ends.

We have here an intriguing but superficial glimpse of the body's program of chemical regulation. Hidden from view is the intricate process of synthesis taking place inside the cells where hormones are made. Equally hidden is the interaction of hormones with their target cells, which receive the messages and then decode them into a series of chemical reactions. Hormones are made in glands and they are heading for target cells, not exactly knowing where they are going, just feeling their way along. The destination of each hormone, however, is predetermined and limited to those cells with specific receptors for that hormone. There is a lock-and-key intimacy that determines which hormones will interact with which cells.

At any one time there are hundreds of messengers circulating around in the bloodstream. With this kind of heavy traffic one could expect plenty of trouble, like a pile-up at the off-ramp, or perhaps a trailer wedged under an overpass. The system, honed by 3 billion years of natural selection, is, however, remarkably free of error. The hormones act only where they have receptors and nowhere else; so while thyroid-stimulating hormone (TSH) is busy binding to cells in the thyroid gland, prompting them to make thyroxine, luteinizing hormone (LH) from the pituitary is stimulating Leydig cells in the testes to make testosterone. Hormones tend not to get in each other's way. Occasionally things go wrong: Boys turn out to look like girls, because the testosterone receptors don't work, or diabetes develops because not enough insulin is present. But on the whole the system is marvelously coordinated to bring together many of the body's separate metabolic activities.

The human body is not the kind of structure that would be described as an engineering masterpiece—there has been no overall plan or plot to its unfolding. The evolutionary process, as François Jacob correctly describes it, is more akin to tinkering than to engineering. Whereas the engineer assembles projects by using specific raw materials and precision tools according to an exact plan, the tinkerer slaps things together from whatever scraps and leftovers are lying around. In this way the hormones, neurotransmitters, and other chemical messengers now present in higher organisms may have been adapted from similar structures in lower organisms where they were most likely utilized for entirely different purposes. There is an economy and continuity here that suggest a tinkerer is at work, pasting things together from evolutionary odds and ends, allowing cells to signal each other with chemical messengers for their mutual benefit.

From Soup to Messengers

The earth first formed from the solar system primordial dust cloud about 4.5 billion years ago, and the first organisms—primitive anaerobic bacteria—appeared about 3.5 billion years ago, leaving an evolutionary gap of 1 billion years for life to be created from nonliving inorganic matter and organic matter. Almost nothing is known about this wondrous creation, but some broad outlines have come into view. The primitive oceans and atmosphere, the setting for the origin of life on earth, bore little resemblance to today's counterparts. For example, there was little oxygen in the primitive atmosphere, which consisted largely of nitrogen, hydrogen, carbon dioxide, ammonia, water, hydrogen sulfide, methane, and probably other simple substances. That life could have evolved from this nonliving matter in this primitive atmosphere was first proposed in the 1920s by Haldane and Oparin. Ultraviolet radiation from the sun could easily have penetrated to the earth's surface to provide the energy necessary for synthetic chemical reactions. In the 1950s, Miller and Urey demonstrated in their laboratory that sparks discharged into gaseous mixtures containing hydrogen, ammonia, methane, and water could produce a host of organic molecules, including amino acids, which are the building blocks of peptide hormones and other proteins. It does not take a giant leap of the imagination to infer from this kind of experiment that the primitive oceans evolved into what is called a "Haldane soup," a body of fluid teeming with basic building blocks—amino acids, nucleotides, and other simple organic molecules from which the first organisms could be constructed. Thus, chemical evolution had to precede biological evolution; simple molecules had to congregate into the complex molecules of living structures. For those of you who are unnerved by the suggestion that you and your ancestors evolved out of a large bowl of soup, a rival theory has recently become available for your consideration—we have evolved from crystal genes in a matrix of clay!

It is a long step from the formation of a Haldane soup consisting of simple organic molecules to the creation of the first primitive single-cell organisms. Ultimately, over the first billion years the first cells emerged out of the Haldane soup and set the stage for natural selection to operate. Over the next 3.5 billion years, more sophisticated, highly efficient organisms were created through a continuous evolutionary process. Gradually, across the abyss of time, a genetic code was established in the form of deoxyribonucleic acid (DNA), a code distinguished by two fundamental characteristics: It could replicate itself accurately, and it could be translated by adaptor molecules into peptides. Chemical messengers became necessary to coordinate the activities of cell clusters. It is these messengers and their role in coordinating the functions of many disparate cell systems in higher organisms, including humans, that will be our major focus of interest.

Across the chasm of evolutionary time, the human body has slowly been assembled from the first single-cell organisms into a biochemical wonder and complexity that is still mostly mysterious. In the course of this evolutionary process, two major networks of interior communication have arisen, the endocrine system and the nervous system, which are jointly responsible for coordinating the intimate relationship among various regions of the body. Both systems rely on chemical messengers to fulfill this life-preserving function.

These two major control networks evolved to maintain body equilibrium by compensating for changes from without and within and by keeping things moving in the right direction. The nervous system uses a set of chemical messengers called neurotransmitters, molecular signals that travel from one nerve cell to the next. Neurotransmitters, for example norepinephrine and acetylcholine, are synthesized inside of nerve cells and are released from each nerve cell when its electrical impulse reaches the next cell. The neurotransmitter then travels across the narrow junction between cells and binds to receptors on the neighboring cell, which then discharges its electrical impulse.

The endrocrine system is composed of a set of cells organized into glands and cell clusters that release chemical messengers called hormones into the bloodstream, where they circulate throughout the body to selected locations to do their work. The hormones are long-range messengers reaching out from one region of the body to perform a vital function at some other distant site.

There is similarity, then, between the endocrine system and the nervous system: Both use chemical messengers and receptors to transmit information from one cell to another cell, and they act in concert to regulate various processes in the body (see Figure 1-1). Both systems work to preserve the harmony of organisms in the face of changes in the environment. The endocrine system acts slowly since its messengers are delivered by the circulatory system, while the nervous system has very rapid response times. Together the two systems coordinate the activities of all body functions.

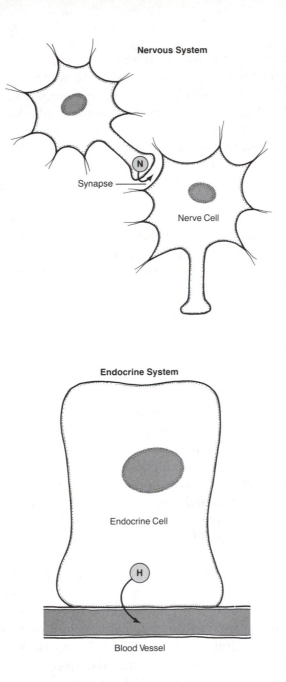

Figure 1-1. Both the endocrine system and the nervous system utilize chemical messengers. Endocrine cells secrete hormones (H) into the circulation to act at distant sites while nerve cells secrete neurotransmitters (N) into the synapse between cells where they act on the neighboring nerve cell.

Today we identify many of these messengers, hormones and neurotransmitters alike, as peptides—that is, simple molecules composed of a linear sequence of amino acids. These peptide messengers are put together inside of cells and the recipes are contained in the genetic code, an instructional program residing in the cells' own DNA. The way the nucleotides are lined up in the DNA determines how the amino acids are lined up in the peptides synthesized within the cells. Each different peptide corresponds to a particular gene coded into DNA.

When were the genes for peptide hormones first programmed into the genetic code, and for what purpose? We don't yet know either what primitive genetic codes looked like or what primitive cells were like, because they are now extinct, replaced by more sophisticated present day versions. We can, however, venture some speculation on these matters. In the more than 4 billion years during which the panorama of chemical and biological evolution on earth has played itself out, nearly 500 million species of organisms have come and gone, leaving about 1 million species now in existence—survivors of an arduous process of natural selection begun long ago. Humans have many biochemical attributes in common with these other survivors, including a universal genetic code and many very similar metabolic pathways and closely related enzymes.

It took thousands of years of inquiry into the function of the human body to discover the existence of hormones and other chemical messengers. The story starts in antiquity with the Greek theory of body regulation. The Greeks held the view that all things were composed of the four elements—air, water, fire, and earth—and that these combined with the four qualities—dry, moist, hot, and cold—to produce the basic body "humors" of blood, phlegm, yellow bile, and black bile. Health was a matter of balance among these constituents; disease resulted when they got out of kilter. This fourfold view of humoral regulation of body function can be viewed as a primitive forerunner of an endocrine system of control. There was no shortage of clinical observation in antiquity that could have led to an endocrine theory. Castrates are a case in point: The removal of the testes of a young male leads to a loss of sexual potency, libido, muscle strength, and the male hair pattern. Castrates were well known throughout the ages, but the idea that the testes secreted an important substance like testosterone that preserved maleness did not arise until much later.

Accurate knowledge about the anatomy of the human body slowly accumulated, including an awareness of the major glands: the pituitary, thyroid, parathyroids, pancreas, adrenals, ovaries, and testes. But their function, although the subject of considerable speculation, not to say imaginative guesswork, remained a mystery. While physicians were busy making astute observations of the clinical syndromes that result from glandular diseases (cretinism, myxedema, hyperthyroidism, adrenal insufficiency, diabetes, tetany, and acromegaly) physiologists were trying to figure out what was going on at a more fundamental level. From their investigations throughout the nineteenth century a consensus slowly emerged—that endocrine glands discharge secretions into the bloodstream, and that these secretions regulate physiologic events throughout the body.

The Theory of Internal Secretions

The French physiologist Claude Bernard first introduced the term "internal secretion" in 1855 in describing the physiology of the liver. There the sugar glucose is synthesized and secreted internally into the bloodstream to help maintain the blood sugar concentration at an adequate level during a prolonged fast. The concept of an *internal* secretion, which is delivered into the bloodstream to circulate throughout the body, is to be distinguished from the concept of an *external* secretion, which is secreted to regions outside of the bloodstream, such as sweat from sweat glands, or pancreas enzymes into the intestine. (The pancreas gland also secretes the hormones insulin and glucagon internally into the bloodstream, where they circulate around the body to regulate sugar metabolism.)

The notion that internal secretions arise from various glands and other organs of the body did not really catch on until the English physiologist Edward Schaefer published his landmark paper on the subject in 1895. Schaefer pointed out that dogs developed diabetes when their pancreas gland was removed and that diabetes could be prevented by pancreatic grafts; he concluded that the pancreas must be secreting something into the blood that prevents the excessive formation of sugar in the blood and urine. He also conjectured, on the basis of the observation that thyroid extracts could prevent myxedema in animals and humans, that the thyroid gland produced an internal secretion. With the theory of internal secretions, the stage was set for the revolutionary advances in hormone physiology and biochemistry that occurred in the twentieth century.

It is a long road from speculation about glands secreting substances into the bloodstream to our present comprehensive understanding of hormone physiology. First, a sensitive test has to be developed to detect a hormone, or else its existence remains mere speculation. Extracts from the secreting organ have to be prepared—and prepared meticulously, so all of the substance you are looking for is not lost or damaged in the process—and this is just the beginning. With an extract and an assay in hand, you are ready to begin the search; you must then proceed to try to isolate the hormone in a pure form. Then, if your chemistry is up to the task, you can identify the chemical structure of the hormone and reproduce it from scratch in the laboratory. Now you are poised to study how and where the hormone works, how it binds to receptors and stimulates cells elsewhere in the body to perform their biochemical tasks.

Endocrinology was launched into a legitimate scientific arena by epinephrine, the first hormone to be isolated and synthesized. A large number of investigators worked for ten long years on the task. The first extracts containing epinephrine were isolated from the adrenal glands of various animals in 1894 by Oliver and Schaefer. When injected into the veins of dogs, these extracts produced a remarkable rise in blood pressure and increased the heart contractions: a hormone assay had been found! Now began a long journey of investigation through the twentieth century. Epinephrine was finally isolated and purified in 1901 and three years later was synthesized in the laboratory. Given the primitive facilities then available to biomedical investigators, this was a tremendous achievement.

While the isolation and synthesis of epinephrine was progressing, the existence of a second hormone, secretin, came to light from a most unexpected source, the small intestine. It was already well known that the upper small intestine (the duodenum) received a digestive juice through a duct from the pancreas. This happened whenever food mixed with acidic stomach fluid passed from the stomach into the duodenum and beyond into the neighboring small intestine (the jejunum). It was also known from experiments in dogs that when dilute hydrochloric acid was placed directly in contact with the lining of the duodenum or jejunum, a marked increase of pancreatic juice flowed into the intestine. Acid touching the cells lining the small intestine somehow provoked the pancreas to secrete a digestive fluid through the pancreatic duct into the duodenum.

How, you may ask, did acid in the duodenum signal the pancreas to brew up these digestive juices? It was presumed that the release occurred via a reflex arc of the nervous system connecting the duodenum to the pancreas—a Pavlovian reflex. This was a time when the nervous system was still perceived to be responsible for most of the communication that went on around the body. The elegant experiments of Bayliss and Starling leading to the discovery in 1902 of secretin brought the endocrine system up onto center stage as a communication network that would eventually come to rival the nervous system as a subject for scientific study. We now know that when released from cells lining the intestines into the bloodstream, secretin circulates to the pancreas, where it stimulates pancreatic cells to produce a juice containing digestive enzymes. Consequently, whenever the contents of the stomach, which include hydrochloric acid (HCl) and partially digested food, are propelled into the duodenum, secretin is released into the circulation and the pancreas swings into action.

This important discovery by Bayliss and Starling was witnessed by Martin, who described it in the following words:

> I happened to be present at their discovery. In an anesthetized dog, a loop of jejunum was tied at its ends and the nerves supplying it dissected out and divided so that it was connected with the rest of the body only by the blood vessels. On the introduction of some weak HCl into the duodenum, secretion from the pancreas occurred and continued for some minutes. After this had subsided a few cubic centimeters of acid were introduced into the enervated loop of jejunum. To our surprise a similarly marked secretion was produced. I remember Starling saying, "Then it must be a chemical reflex." Rapidly cutting off a further piece of jejunum he rubbed its mucous membrane with sand in weak HCl, filtered and injected it into the jugular vein of the animal. After a few moments the pancreas responded by a much greater secretion than had occurred before. It was a great afternoon.

Another 65 years went by before pure secretin was finally isolated and shown to be a small peptide composed of 27 amino acids. Major advances in protein chemistry were necessary before the structure of

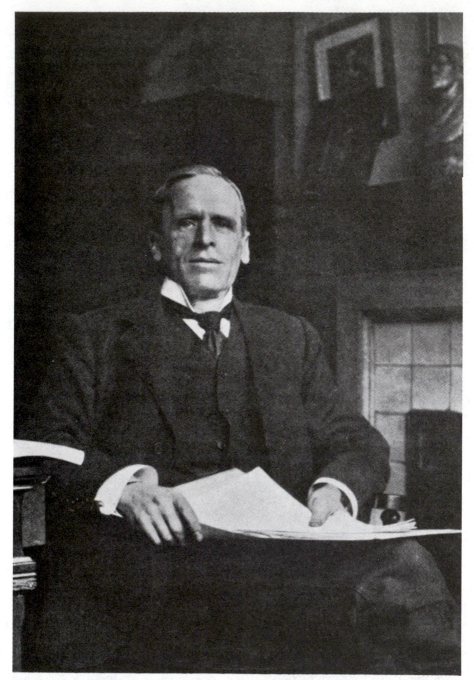

Ernest Henry Starling first introduced the word "hormone" in 1905 to describe circulating chemical messengers.

secretin and many other peptide chemical messengers could be determined.

Not long after his discovery of secretin, Starling first introduced the word "hormone" in a 1905 lecture entitled "The Chemical Correlation of the Functions of the Body." This important lecture expanded Schaefer's ideas on internal secretions and developed the concept that hormones could be produced in certain regions of the body to circulate in the bloodstream as chemical messengers to other regions, where they act at specific target sites to regulate the metabolic needs of the whole organism. "Hormone" is derived from the Greek verb *hormao*, meaning to excite or arouse. Thus a hormone is a substance that sets into motion a set of metabolic events that would otherwise lie dormant. Hormones arouse our metabolic machinery to perform at an optimum level for the tasks at hand. All the hormones together form a network called the endocrine system, and the study of this system and its disorders is called endocrinology. Building on the work of Schaefer and other investigators of the nineteenth century, Starling set this new discipline in motion.

The discovery, purification, and synthesis of epinephrine and secretin illustrate a process that has been repeated over and over again for many different hormones throughout the twentieth century. Extracts are prepared from a gland or an organ and a biological assay (a method for detecting the presence of a specific hormone) is developed. The assay is refined and used to guide the purification and isolation steps. After the hormone is isolated in a pure form it can be used for therapy and its chemical structure can be determined.

Occasionally the isolation of a hormone will have a dramatic impact worldwide. The isolation of insulin by Banting and Best and the isolation of the hypothalamic thyrotropin-releasing hormone (TRH) by Schally and Guillemin are major accomplishments that have caught the public eye. But for the most part, the discovery and purification of hormones has proceeded in quiet obscurity behind the scenes, in the world's major research laboratories.

Research into how these hormones work has lagged slightly behind the initial isolation of the hormones themselves but the discoveries have been equally exciting. The first hormone isolated, epinephrine, was also the first hormone for which a biochemical mechanism of action was discovered. Sutherland demonstrated in the 1950s that epinephrine stimulates the synthesis of the second messenger, cyclic adenosine monophosphate (cyclic AMP) inside of liver cells; cyclic AMP then initiates a cascade of biochemical reactions, which results in the production of glucose by the liver cells. The discovery of cyclic AMP was a major scientific breakthrough in understanding how many hormones work. Since Sutherland's key discovery, many different hormones have been shown to act on their target cells through this second messenger, cyclic AMP. The general rule can be stated as follows: When a hormone (like epinephrine) acts at its receptor on the surface of a cell, it initiates a series of chemical reactions that result in the synthesis of cyclic AMP inside the cell; the hormone, acting outside the cell, is considered to be the *first messenger*, while cyclic AMP, acting inside the cell as a catalyst for further chemical reactions, is the *second messenger*. We will consider this important mechanism of hormone action in more detail in the next chapter.

Throughout the first half of the twentieth century, the measurement of hormones gradually improved in sensitivity and accuracy. The initial bioassays, relying on specific biologic effects of hormones, gradually gave way to more sensitive bioassays and chemical assays as the hormones were purified and their structure determined. By the 1950s many more hormones had been isolated and numerous assays devised to detect them in the bloodstream. The situation was by no means optimal; many of these assays were cumbersome, technically difficult, and too insensitive to detect normal blood levels of many hormones. Nevertheless, they were good enough to establish a comprehensive view of the endocrine system, which can be summarized as follows: Hormones are made by specific cells in specific organs of vertebrates and are released into the circulation, where they are carried to target sites throughout the body.

Now, many extracts, assays, isolations, and syntheses later, we sit on a mountain of knowledge about many different hormones. The effort exerted to secure this knowledge has been enormous and so has the benefit to mankind. Previously lethal and debilitating diseases like diabetes, cretinism, myxedema, adrenal failure, pituitary insufficiency, and many other disorders of the endocrine system have all been brought under control. Indeed, the field of endocrinology now rivals the field of infectious diseases in its ability to treat disease, and for a similar reason—both are built on a bedrock of over a hundred years of tough, painstaking scientific research, the byproduct of which has been a series of exceedingly useful therapeutic interventions. In light of this progress, the present national retreat from the education of our children in science and from support for basic research can only be viewed as sheer folly, a disintegration at the core of a once vigorous society, now surging forth into a world of space weapons, home videos, and hot tubs.

On the horizon of these accomplishments lay new assays that would consolidate classical notions of hormone physiology and lead not only to a radically new view of the duality of endocrine and nervous communication systems but also to a total reformulation of our notions about the evolutionary origins of hormones and other chemical messengers.

Modern Concepts

It took several thousand years of inquiry into the function of the human body to discover the existence of hormones and other chemical messengers. The classical view that hormones are made by specialized cells in specific regions of the body, where they are released into the bloodstream and transported to distant target sites, was methodically pieced together over 100 years by thousands of investigators. This view included the notion that hormones were unique to higher organisms and were necessary to coordinate the many diverse physiologic events occurring in these complex organisms.

This classical view has recently undergone a major upheaval. The hormone systems have turned out to be considerably more complex than originally envisioned, resembling a youth soccer game even more than a congested freeway of traffic. Hormones have been discovered in obscure regions in the human body where they were never supposed to be, as well as in lower organisms, where their role still remains to be defined. These startling discoveries have shaken the foundations of hormone physiology and have reshuffled the concepts about chemical messengers.

The detection of hormones in places where they weren't supposed to be was the result of a giant step forward in assay sensitivity, not unlike a Galilean telescope pushing the thinking out toward the moons of Jupiter. The time was ripe for the development of a sensitive hormone assay in the 1950s: The groundwork had been laid in physics and immunology; radioisotopes had been discovered and enthusiastically applied to the study of biological systems, and the interaction between antibodies and antigens was already reasonably well understood. Such a radioimmunoassay is basically quite simple. The radiolabeled hormone interacts with a specific antibody to form a bound complex. The amount of radioactivity that is bound in the complex is a measure of the affinity between the antibody and the radiolabeled hormone. Unlabeled hormone added to the picture competes with radiolabeled hormone for antibody binding sites and causes a fall in the amount of radioactivity in the bound complex.

Berson and Yalow developed this assay to measure plasma insulin concentrations in diabetics and normal persons. They injected beef insulin into guinea pigs, which produced antibodies against the insulin. They then labeled pure beef insulin with radioiodine (I^{131}) and, using the I^{131}-insulin and the guinea pig antibodies against insulin, they were able to measure accurately the insulin concentrations in human plasma.

Their assay has opened up whole new vistas of inquiry. The explosion of hormone research following its introduction has been remarkable. Radioimmunoassays have now been developed for many different hormones. The exquisite sensitivity and specificity of the method allows it to be used on very small samples of plasma and tissue extracts; multiple samples of plasma with low hormone concentrations can be processed quickly. Nothing could be more ideal to probe the intricacies of biological systems.

Hormones previously thought to be made in specific organs have now been discovered all over the place. The pancreatic hormone, insulin, has been found in brain cells; the hypothalamic hormone, somatostatin, has been discovered in the pancreas and gut; the intestinal hormones gastrin and cholecystokinin have been found in the central nervous system, where they presumably act as neurotransmitters! Quite surprisingly, many cancerous tumors have been found to secrete a variety of hormones into the bloodstream. Hormones everywhere, with no end in sight to the new discoveries.

Most exciting of all has been the recent discovery of peptide hormones in lower invertebrate organisms. Jesse Roth and his colleagues at the National Institutes of Health, by using a variety of insulin assays, have discovered substances similar to insulin in fruit flies, earthworms, protozoa, and fungi; and they have discovered the hormones somatostatin and adrenocorticotropic hormone (ACTH) in protozoa. Other investigators have also found hormones in lower organisms, so these findings seem to be on fairly solid ground. Much more work needs to be done, however, to demonstrate conclusively that insulin and other hormones found in microorganisms are similar or identical to the hormones in humans.

The discovery of peptide hormones in unicellular organisms as well as in different locations in the human body has momentous implications for unraveling the evolution of chemical messengers. On the basis of these data Roth has proposed that the endocrine system and the nervous system have evolved from a common ancestral system in which chemical messengers were employed by primitive cells as signals to neighboring cells. Because these messengers must have conveyed some selective advantage in terms of growth or acquisition of nutrients from the primitive environment, they have been highly conserved. In the course of evolution, more complex organisms eventually adopted some of these primitive messengers as hormones, neurotransmitters, and such other intercellular messengers as tissue growth factors, prostaglandins and interferon. Thus chemical signals between cells began early in evolution, leading ultimately through natural selection to the hormones, pheromones, neurotransmitters, and other chemical messengers of present-day organisms.

This evolution may in part explain the remarkable unity of intercellular communication that has recently come to light. Roth's hypothesis regarding the evolutionary origin of chemical messengers, published in 1982, relies on the detection in present-day bacteria of hormones that originated about 1 billion years ago. These bacteria are very sophisticated organisms compared to their single-cell ancestor organisms, which first appeared on earth approximately 3.5 billion years ago, nearly 1 billion years after the origin of the earth. The modern bacteria, complete with elaborate biochemical machinery, including the ability to make hormonelike substances, have appeared relatively recently on the evolutionary stage.

As we have seen, the endocrine and nervous systems have developed in tandem from similar evolutionary origins, but the plot thickens on deeper probing: When we examine several recent exciting discoveries, we note that some nerve cells make molecules that are secreted into the circulation to act as hormones at distant targets, and some hormones are made in nerve cells where they act as neurotransmitters. During the course of evolution the chemical messengers differentiated into endocrine and nervous systems, and yet there is common ground, shared structures that illustrate a certain unity and economy of nature.

We have so far taken a rather limited view of chemical messengers—hormones and neurotransmitters—that regulate communications between glands, nerve cells, and other cell systems in all higher organisms. But inside of cells are all kinds of chemical messengers: re-

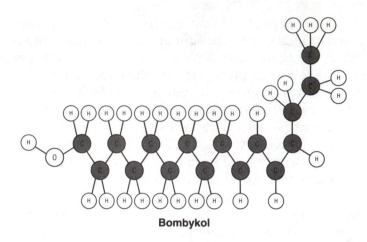

Bombykol

Figure 1-2. Bombykol is a pheromone secreted by the female silk moth. Only several hundred molecules of this chemical messenger are necessary to signal the male silk moth about the presence of a female.

pressors and inducers regulating the genetic code, enzymes regulating various metabolic pathways, and cyclic AMP regulating the enzymes. All hormones exert their influence on cells by stimulating a change in these intracellular messengers.

Many organisms, such as insects and fish, secrete chemical messengers that are received by receptors on other individuals of the same species. These messengers, secreted from glands to the *outside* of the body, are called "pheromones," from the Greek verb *pherein*, meaning to transfer.

Pheromones are potent and highly specific; they are used as sexual attractants, alarm substances, trail guides to food, and territorial markers. Queen bees secrete a pheromone that is ingested by worker bees to prevent them from producing other queen bees. Ants lay down a trail of pheromone to direct other ants to food—when the food is gone no more pheromone is secreted by ants returning to the nest, and the trail evaporates within minutes. The silkworm moth sex attractant, *bombykol*, a small 16-carbon linear molecule, is one of the most potent pheromones yet discovered (see Figure 1-2). Only several hundred molecules per cubic centimeter are necessary to stimulate a male sexual response. The pheromone is volatile; consequently it can be distributed by wind up to a distance of several miles from the female moth. Lewis Thomas in *The Lives of a Cell* has written a vivid description of what it might be like to be a downwind male moth receiving a bombykol sex signal:

> The messages are urgent, but they may arrive, for all we know, in a fragrance of ambiguity. "At home, 4 P.M. today," says the female moth, and releases a brief explosion of bombykol, a single molecule of which will tremble the hairs of any male within miles and send him driving upwind in a confusion of ardor. But it is doubtful if he has an awareness of being caught in an aerosol of chemical attractant. On the contrary, he probably finds suddenly that it has become an excellent day, the weather remarkably bracing, the time appropriate for a bit of exercise of the old wings, a brisk turn upwind. En route, traveling the gradient of bombykol, he notes the presence of other males, heading in the same direction, all in a good mood, inclined to race for the sheer sport of it. Then, when he reaches his destination, it may seem to him the most extraordinary of coincidences, the greatest piece of luck: "Bless my soul, what have we here!"

It is only natural for you to wonder at this point whether or not humans make pheromones. I certainly hope not. There would be plenty of trouble if we were all at the mercy of each other's secretions, the air filled with trail guides and sex attractants driving us upwind, as it were, in a confusion of ardor.

From Bacteria to Humans

Chemical messengers have arisen over eons of evolutionary time. Originating in primitive organisms for unclear purposes, hormones have appeared on the scene to serve ultimately as signals between cells. Evolution, acting in the fashion of a tinkerer, has stacked layer upon layer of change, molding a finely honed endocrine system in higher organisms from the scraps of natural selection. The whole process, an amazingly complex ordeal, has taken well over a billion years.

It was not until late into the nineteenth century that the existence of these hormones was discovered. Since then the development of highly refined hormone assays along with other scientific advances in the fields of biology and chemistry have led to a detailed understanding of hormone structure and action. The discovery of hormones in primitive organisms and in the nervous system of higher organisms has recently opened up new vistas of thinking about the body's regulation by chemical messengers.

The striking biochemical similarity of all present day organisms indicates that they may have originated from a single set of interbreeding organisms. So it is not totally surprising to find hormonelike substances in lower organisms similar to those in higher organisms. As we have seen, the hormones appeared long before they had any business being here and well before we or anything like us showed up on the scene. The hormones had been hanging around in bacteria and fungi, biding their time, probably performing some useful tasks, until they were eventually selected in the course of evolution as specific messengers in higher organisms.

The pheromones are fascinating, as are the neurotransmitters of the nervous system, and the intracellular regulators like cyclic AMP, but to zero in on the orchestration of metabolic activities in the human body we will set aside these important topics and in this book focus directly on the hormones, that multitude of chemical messengers floating around in the circulation. Where in the world are all these hormones coming from, where are they going, and what do they do when they get there? These are the questions we will be unraveling, trying to uncover the various layers of understanding provided by scientific investigation.

2

ON HORMONES
AND OTHER MATTERS

■

*Persons attempting to find a motive in this narrative will be prosecuted;
persons attempting to find a moral in it will be banished; persons attempting
to find a plot in it will be shot.*
　　　　　　　　　—Mark Twain, Introduction to *Huckleberry Finn*

Now we are ready to dig in and try to make sense out of the hormone
systems that have been imposed upon us by the mythical tinkerer.
There is no overall motive or plot here; the various networks of chemical
messengers within the body are loosely bound together by a certain
economy. If you make it through this chapter intact then you are home
free to enjoy a series of intriguing discoveries scattered through the
remainder of the book. If the science gets a little thick, don't panic.
Shift into a skimming mode, ponder a few of the figures, go out for a
jog and come back later to fill in a few of the arduous details. Although
at times you may feel that you are in a briar patch rather than a rose
garden, there is no other way to understand the complexity of our
intricate hormone systems. So settle back, take a long draw on your
favorite beverage, put on a little background music (I would recom-
mend the Brandenburg Concertos for this chapter), and brace yourself
for a brief voyage through the world of hormone physiology.

In humans and other higher organisms, hormones orginate in specific regions of the body, unique places where the cells have specialized, each kind to perform a single function. The specialized cells
have been organized into glands and clusters—like small factories in
Silicon Valley—that make the hormones and then release them into the

circulation. The hormones wind their way through the body to distant locations, where they bind to special receptors at target cells to initiate a cascade of chemical reactions inside the cells. The hormone-manufacturing glands work together in close union, constantly communicating with each other by feedback signals to achieve an optimal metabolic balance throughout the body. This precisely coordinated hormone network is well organized to deal with a wide range of perturbations from the outside world in the interest of survival. Jostle an important body chemical like glucose in the wrong direction and hormones will come roaring out of the woodwork to tenaciously defend the status quo.

The Hormone Factories

The major hormone-producing regions of the human body are depicted in Figure 2-1, which presents what has come to be known as the classical view of the endocrine system, a discrete system of glands and cell clusters organized to control our metabolic needs. The hormones produced by cells located in these regions are secreted directly into the circulation and travel to target cells in other parts of the body. These hormone-producing cell clusters have presumably been located in this way through the course of evolution to maximize their efficiency as regulators of the body's chemistry.

The *hypothalamus* sits in the brain, at the pinnacle of the endocrine system, just above the pituitary gland, rather like a central relay station or perhaps a clearing house, receiving messages from nerve cells elsewhere in the brain and then sending out to the pituitary hormone signals based on these brain messages. There are at least seven different hypothalamic hormones, all of which are peptides; they are dumped directly into a specialized network of blood vessels (the arrow in Figure 2-1) called the *hypothalamic-pituitary portal circulation* that carries the hormones to the pituitary gland, where they stimulate or inhibit the release of pituitary hormones. The hypothalamus, then, is the originator of a set of chemical signals that regulate numerous important glands throughout the body. As a center of control, it receives not only messages from the higher brain via nerve terminals but also hormone feedback signals from the regulated glands.

As an example, consider the regulation of the thyroid gland by the hypothalamus as shown in Figure 2-2. The hypothalamic peptide called thyrotropin-releasing hormone (TRH) finds its way to the pituitary gland; there it induces the release of thyroid-stimulating hor-

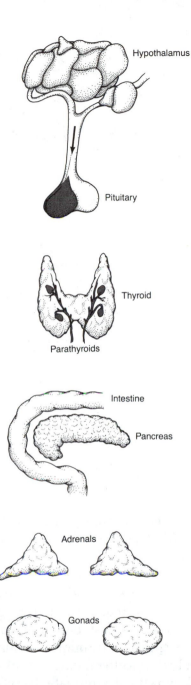

Figure 2-1. The major hormone-producing regions of the human body. All of these structures release hormones into the general circulation except the hypothalamus which releases its hormones into the portal circulation (arrow) connecting the hypothalamus to the pituitary gland.

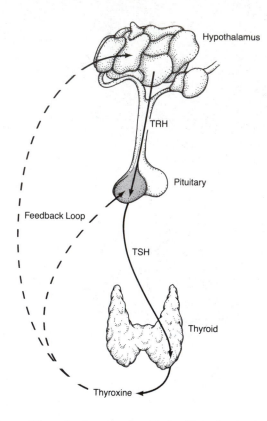

Hypothalamus

TRH

Pituitary

Feedback Loop

TSH

Thyroid

Thyroxine

Figure 2-2. The release of thyroxine from the thyroid gland into the circulation results from the stimulation of the thyroid by TSH, which itself is released from the pituitary by the hypothalamic hormone TRH. The feedback loop (dashed line) regulates the production of these hormones. Similar cascades occur for the adrenals and gonads.

mone (TSH), which travels through the bloodstream to its receptors on cells in the thyroid gland, stimulating the thyroid to release thyroxine to regulate the body's metabolism. The increased blood level of thyroxine in turn inhibits the further production of TRH and TSH, so that the TRH/TSH/thyroxine cascade is tightly regulated at an optimum set point. Suppose that your thyroid glands decided to quit making thyroxine one day—to sit back and watch the show while the rest of your body is churning through its usual metabolic paces. The hypothalamus will react to the falling serum thyroxine level by producing more TRH, which will stimulate the pituitary to produce more TSH, and the TSH will act directly on the thyroid gland, stimulating it to restore the serum thyroxine level back to normal. Similar finely tuned cascades also occur from the hypothalamus to the adrenal glands and the gonads (ovaries in women and testes in men).

The *pituitary gland*, located at the base of the brain just beneath the hypothalamus, is divided into two major regions, front and back (or *anterior* and *posterior*). An intriguing gland, it is the locale for the second stage in the flow of chemical information through the hypothalamic-pituitary-glandular cascade. The anterior part of the pituitary gland secretes into the bloodstream six peptide hormones that control a broad spectrum of metabolic events, as shown in Table 2-1 (the pituitary gland also produces some other interesting peptides, such as β-endorphin and dynorphin, for which no function is yet known). It is easy to see that any major disturbance of the hypothalamus or pituitary gland from disease or trauma can wreak havoc in the body's metabolic economy and lead to serious disability.

The *thyroid gland* is shaped like a shield (its name derives from the Greek word *thyreos*, meaning "shield") and lies just below the Adam's apple in the front of the neck. It makes several hormones, including thyroxine, which control the metabolic rate of many different cells throughout the body. As we have seen, the thyroid itself is regulated by TSH from the pituitary, so that the blood level of thyroxine is tightly controlled within a narrow range.

The *parathyroids* are a set of four small glands located in the neck, right next to the thyroid gland. They regulate the blood calcium level by secreting parathyroid hormone (PTH) into the bloodstream. PTH promotes the absorption of calcium in the diet by the small intestine, the release of calcium from bones, and the conservation of calcium by the kidneys. Be prepared for a bad case of tetany if your parathyroid glands stop making PTH and your serum calcium level falls. Get ready for bone pain and kidney stones if your parathyroid glands produce too much PTH.

Hormones made in the pancreas and the gut regulate the digestion and utilization of foods. When the contents of the stomach are propelled into the small intestine these hormones are released into the bloodstream. Insulin and glucagon from the pancreas are responsible for regulating the metabolism of carbohydrates, proteins, and fats. When insulin is not made in adequate amounts or does not work properly at its receptors, the disease diabetes mellitus occurs. Similarly, digestive juices from the gall bladder and pancreas are excreted into the gut by hormones (like secretin and cholecystokinin) originating from the cells lining the gut. These hormones from the gut and pan-

TABLE 2-1

The Hormones and Their Functions

Origin	Hormones	Function
Hypothalamus	Stimulators	Pituitary Hormone Regulation
	Inhibitors	
Pituitary, Anterior	ACTH	Adrenal Control
	FSH	Gonad Regulation
	GH	Growth Stimulation
	LH	Gonad Regulation
	Prolactin	Breast Milk Production
	TSH	Thyroid Control
Pituitary, Posterior	ADH	Water Conservation
	Oxytocin	Uterus Contraction and Breast Milk Excretion
Thyroid	Thyroxine	Metabolic Rate Control
Parathyroid	PTH	Calcium Regulation
Gut	Gut Hormones	Food Digestion
Pancreas	Insulin	Glucose Metabolism
	Glucagon	
Adrenals	Cortisol	Body Preservation
	Aldosterone	Salt Conservation
	Epinephrine	Stress Response
Ovaries	Estradiol	Female Characteristics
	Progesterone	
Testes	Testosterone	Male Characteristics

creas provide the coordination of digestive events so that we can assimilate a wide variety of foodstuffs.

There are two *adrenal glands*, one located just above each kidney. Their importance in the maintenance of life was not known until the middle of the nineteenth century, when Thomas Addison discovered that profound debility in humans can result from disease of the adrenals, while others demonstrated the same effect in animals. Each adrenal gland is composed of two parts: an inner core called the *medulla*, which secretes the hormone epinephrine, and an outer shell called the *cortex*, which produces the steroid hormones cortisol and aldosterone as well as several other substances.

Cortisol acts on many different cells in the body to preserve appetite, blood pressure, and nutritional well-being. It is controlled by the pituitary hormone, adrenocorticotropic hormone (ACTH), which in turn is regulated by corticotropin-releasing hormone (CRH) from the hypothalamus. The three hormones CRH/ACTH/cortisol form a regulatory cascade, complete with feedback inhibition designed to keep the concentration of cortisol in the bloodstream at an optimal level.

The other major adrenal cortex hormone, aldosterone, acts at the kidney and several other sites to conserve salt and, by doing so, to regulate the blood pressure. Because aldosterone also acts to stimulate the kidney to secrete potassium into the urine, when aldosterone is deficient not only does the blood pressure fall, but the serum potassium may rise to a dangerous level.

The *adrenal medulla*, or inner core, releases epinephrine under conditions of stress. Epinephrine acts on the heart, lungs, and blood vessels to increase the circulation of nutrients and oxygen to other organs; it also increases the production of such metabolic fuels as glucose and fatty acids. Epinephrine is an emergency hormone used by the body (along with several others) to stimulate rapid deployment of fuels—a hormone for all seasons waiting in the wings in case there is trouble.

The *gonads* are responsible for reproduction; they are concerned with survival of the species rather than survival of the individual. Like the thyroid and adrenal glands, the gonads are under control of the hypothalamus and the pituitary through a cascade of regulatory hormones. The gonads produce two important products: the germ cells that unite to form new life, and the sex hormones that enhance germ cell maturation, mating, and uterus reception of an embryo. The ovaries produce the hormones estradiol and progesterone. Under cyclic pituitary control, these regulate the menstrual cycle and release of eggs into the fallopian tubes; estradiol also acts to preserve female sex characteristics. Testosterone, produced by the testes, is responsible for male development in fetal life and at puberty; it controls male libido and potency, adult male sexual characteristics, and the development of spermatozoa in the follicle cells of the testes.

Table 2-1 presents a summary of the hormones originating from the major endocrine systems throughout the body. There is some coherence here, with feedback regulation between the pituitary and its target organs, as well as an inherent coordination of other hormones concerned with nutrient digestion and metabolism. In this classical view, specialized cells are organized into glands and clusters to secrete hormones into the circulation to act at different sites. It is not the whole story, as we have seen in Chapter 1, for some of these hormones are produced in other places (such as the brain and cancer cells) and nobody yet knows what they are doing there. It is important to understand the traditional view, if only to have a framework for understanding the conceptual changes that are sure to come and those that are already emerging. For example, other chemical messengers known to be located in the pituitary, central brain, and gut are not included in the classical picture because they cannot yet be shown to fit in.

At present we know that there are two major types of hormones in the body, *peptides* and *steroids*, different from each other in how they are made, what they are made of, and how they act at target sites. The peptide hormones are composed of *amino acids* strung together in a linear sequence. These peptides bind to their receptors on the *surface* of target cells and promote chemical reactions inside of the cells via second messengers. In contrast, the steroid hormones are made from *cholesterol* in a characteristic ring structure (see Figure 2-3). These steroids bind to receptors *inside* of cells and are then transported into the cell nucleus; there they act by regulation of the genetic code programmed into DNA. The peptides and steroids together form an integral network of regulation throughout the body. It is important to have a clear understanding of how these two sets of hormones are synthesized and how they act at their target sites.

The Synthesis of Peptide Hormones

Twenty amino acids are specified by the genetic code. Since the code is universal, all plant and animal proteins found in nature are composed of some combination of these same amino acids. Peptides are molecules that contain two or more amino acids linked to each other by a special chemical bond; proteins are simply large peptides. The peptide hormones (those hormones composed of amino acids) come in all shapes and sizes: TRH contains 3 amino acids, ACTH contains 39 amino acids, and PTH contains 84 amino acids. The cells that synthesize these peptide hormones contain a genetic code in the DNA nucleotide sequence that specifies the amino acid sequence for each hormone. In other words, the nucleotide sequence in DNA codes for the amino acid sequence in peptide hormones.

The synthesis of a peptide hormone begins in the nucleus of a cell (see Figure 2-4). The code for the hormone is transcribed from DNA to a long strand of nuclear ribonucleic acid (nRNA) and this strand is then modified to messenger ribonucleic acid (mRNA) by an enzyme that splices off unneeded information. The mRNA is transferred from the nucleus to the cell cytoplasm, where the hormone code (now contained in mRNA) is translated into a peptide chain. The growing

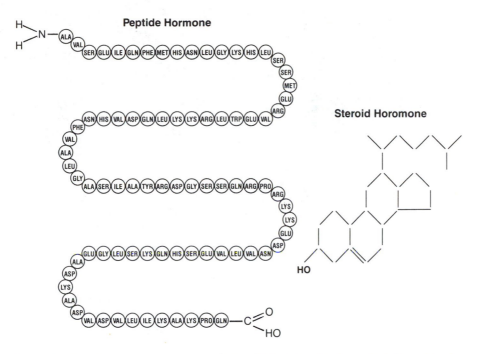

Figure 2-3. Peptide hormones are composed of a linear array of amino acids held together by peptide bonds. Shown here is the 84-amino-acid parathyroid hormone which maintains calcium balance in the blood. Steroid hormones are all derived from cholesterol and contain the charactersitic four ring structure.

peptide chain passes through the membrane of a little cytoplasmic saccule that is transported to other regions of the cell. At this point the peptide is too long, containing an ill-fated segment at one end. When that is clipped off by enzymes, what is left is the final version of the hormone.

The initial long peptide chain is called a _preprohormone_; the "pre" region is a short strand of amino acids responsible for getting the peptide into the saccule; when its job is accomplished it is clipped off, discarded, like a piece of excess baggage, onto the cell's metabolic scrap heap. The "pro" region is also clipped off, and the peptide hormone is finally packaged into storage granules, where it will reside until the time is ripe to release the hormone, through the plasma membrane, into the circulation. The whole process is illustrated in Figure 2-4 for the peptide parathyroid hormone (PTH), which is released into the circulation from parathyroid cells when the serum calcium level falls below normal. The PTH circulates to the bones and

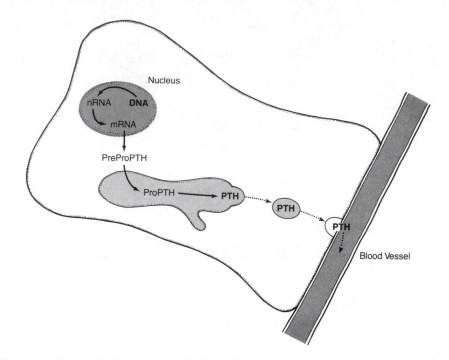

Figure 2-4. The synthesis, storage, and release of parathyroid hormone in parathyroid gland cells in the neck. Release and synthesis are regulated by the serum calcium level.

kidneys, releasing calcium from the bones and reabsorbing calcium from the urine, as well as promoting the formation of active vitamin D to increase calcium absorption from the small intestine. All of these processes act in concert to raise the serum calcium level back to normal. At this point, the secretory granules in the parathyroid cells get the message to quit releasing the PTH. This is feedback regulation at its best, keeping the serum calcium level right where it belongs, so that the heart cells, muscle cells, and many other cells that rely on a normal serum calcium level can function properly.

Now, as you reel back and grasp at the complexity of peptide hormone synthesizing process, you might wonder: Why all the elaborate machinery involving countless enzymes and transfer processes, most of which have only recently been discovered? Why the intricate transfer of information from DNA to nRNA to mRNA? Why the preprohormone, the prohormone, the saccules, and the secretory granules? Three billion years of natural selection to arrive at a process where a hundred things can go wrong? The answers to these questions will have to await further research on the regulation of peptide hormone synthesis.

Almost nothing is known at present about how a falling calcium level in the serum signals the parathyroid cells to release PTH from secretory granules and to synthesize new PTH starting from the DNA code. We are similarly ignorant about how changes in the serum glucose level regulate insulin and glucagon synthesis.

The large peptide hormones that are made in the pituitary, parathyroids, gut, and pancreas are probably all produced by this complex type of synthetic process, and much more needs to be learned about the details of regulation. About the synthesis of the very small peptide hormones produced in the hypothalamus little is known at present.

The Action of Peptide Hormones

Released into the bloodstream from their cells of origin, the peptide hormones circulate throughout the body, meandering through capillaries in search of specific target cells, where they will initiate important chemical reactions—LH in search of Leydig cells in the testes, ACTH in search of adrenal cortex cells, PTH in search of bone and kidney cells, and insulin in search of liver, fat, and muscle cells. How does a peptide hormone recognize a target cell or, conversely, how does the target cell recognize a specific hormone? Figure 2-5 gives a schematic view of the recognition process. All target cells in the body have a surface envelope called a *plasma membrane* separating the exterior environment from the inside of the cell, which is composed of *cytoplasm* and a *nucleus*. The cytoplasm contains practically all of the metabolic machinery of the cells, including many enzymes, mitochondria, endoplasmic reticulum, golgi complexes, lysosomes, and a number of important nutrients. The nucleus is surrounded by its own envelope, the *nuclear membrane*, and contains the cell's DNA, as well as proteins and enzymes that are responsible for regulating and transcribing the genetic code. Peptide hormones are recognized by specific receptor molecules embedded in the plasma membrane on the surface of target cells. Hormone and receptor fit together like a lock and key.

The blood is filled with many different hormones at low concentration, and from this dilute mixture each is selected by target cells with specific surface receptors. Nature has evolved hormones and their receptors in tandem to carry out long-distance chemical communication throughout the body. Peptide hormone receptors have several unique properties that enable them to function as extremely efficient hormone detectors. First of all, they are highly specific, so that they bind to just the right hormone—TSH receptors on the surface of

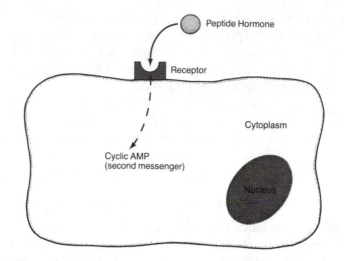

Peptide Hormone

Receptor

Cytoplasm

Cyclic AMP
(second messenger)

Nucleus

Figure 2-5. Interaction of a peptide hormone with a target cell receptor to produce the intracellular second messenger cyclic AMP occurs at the cell surface.

thyroid cells bind only to TSH, letting other peptide hormones pass them by; ACTH receptors on adrenal cortex cells bind only to ACTH. Secondly, receptors have a very high binding affinity for their corresponding hormone; this is essential because of the very low concentration of peptide hormones in the blood.

What happens after a peptide hormone binds to its receptor on the surface of a target cell? How does such a hormone, binding to the *surface* of a target cell, set in motion a chain of chemical reactions *inside* the cell? An answer to these important questions was first provided by Sutherland and his co-workers in the 1950s while they were investigating the mechanism of action of glucagon and epinephrine.

They discovered a new substance inside of liver cells called cyclic adenosine monophosphate (cyclic AMP) and were able to show that cyclic AMP accumulated in the cells when cells were exposed to epinephrine and glucagon. Further studies showed that cyclic AMP was synthesized from adenosine triphosphate (ATP) in a chemical reaction catalyzed by adenylate cyclase, an enzyme that resides in the plasma membrane, or envelope, of the cell and is activated when epinephrine or glucagon binds to its specific receptors. Sutherland therefore surmised that the hormones act at the surface of the cell, setting in motion the activation of adenylate cyclase and the synthesis of cyclic AMP inside the cell, whereupon the cyclic AMP then proceeds to promote a whole series of chemical reactions in the cell cytoplasm. Cyclic AMP was designated as a "second messenger" to distinguish it from those hormones (the "first messengers") which act at the cell surface and initiate the synthesis of cyclic AMP inside of the cell.

Cyclic AMP has subsequently been discovered in many cells throughout the body and in many organisms throughout the evolutionary ladder, including some bacteria. The discovery of cyclic AMP by Sutherland opened the door for a multitude of studies, which have led, as we shall see, to a detailed understanding of how peptide hormones work. But there are several peptide hormones—insulin, prolactin, and growth hormone—that do not utilize cyclic AMP as a second messenger. The discovery of the second messenger for these hormones should open up a whole new layer of our understanding of hormone action in the future.

Steroid Hormones

Steroids are a breed of hormones considerably different from peptides. In general they are much smaller than peptides and can wander into and out of cells almost at their leisure, although they can be trapped inside of their target cells by high-affinity steroid receptor molecules. Of all the hormones shown in Table 2-1 only those made in the adrenals, ovaries, and testes are steroids. The steroid hormones, cortisol and aldosterone, are produced by cells in the adrenal cortex; estradiol and progesterone are made by interstitial cells in the ovaries; and testosterone is made by Leydig cells in the testes.

The starting point for the synthesis of steroid hormones is cholesterol, which is stored inside fat droplets in the cell cytoplasm. Cholesterol is processed by enzymes through a series of steps (depicted in Figure 2-6) leading to its end product, steroid hormones. The key intermediate substance in these reactions is pregnenolone, from which the adrenal steroids and sex steroids are derived. The conversion of cholesterol to pregnenolone is the rate-controlling step in the steroid cascade and is regulated by chemical messengers from the pituitary. But the enzymes necessary for the next step, the processing of pregnenolone to cortisol and aldosterone, are located in the adrenal cortex cells; and the enzymes leading to the synthesis of testosterone and estradiol are located in the testes and ovaries.

Interestingly, peptide and steroid hormones can and do regulate the synthesis of each other. The output of steroid hormones from the adrenals and gonads is regulated by peptide hormones from the pituitary. For example, the synthesis of cortisol (a steroid) in adrenal

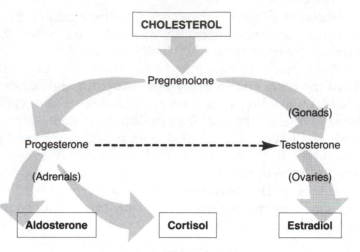

Figure 2-6. Synthesis of principle steroid hormones from cholesterol occurs inside of specialized cells in the adrenals and gonads.

cells is markedly increased by ACTH (a peptide) from the pituitary. ACTH binds to plasma membrane receptors on the adrenal cells, causing a release of cyclic AMP inside the cells. Acting as a second messenger, cyclic AMP in adrenal cells activates key enzymes that increase the production of pregnenolone from cholesterol and consequently increase the output of cortisol.

By a similar mechanism, the pituitary peptide hormone LH promotes an increased output of testosterone from the testes and estradiol from the ovaries. By feedback inhibition, rising serum levels of cortisol, testosterone, and estradiol directly suppress the pituitary output of ACTH and LH and probably suppress the hypothalamic-releasing hormones for ACTH and LH.

Not only are steroid and peptide hormones synthesized by entirely different pathways in their cells of origin, but their action at target cells also occurs by different mechanisms. Steroids, to repeat, do not bind to cell surface receptors but rather enter cells freely and are then bound in the cytoplasm by receptors. The steroid-receptor complex then migrates into the cell nucleus and attaches itself there to specific regions of DNA. This interaction unhinges a piece of the genetic code into a specific messenger RNA (mRNA), which eventually gives rise to the production of protein in the cytoplasm. Steroids increase the cellular synthesis of specific proteins, so that the metabolism of the target cells is altered. Peptides operate differently. Their action leads via cyclic

AMP to alteration of proteins already present in the target cell. With steroids, new proteins are made, but with peptides, existing inactive proteins (enzymes) are activated. Since the activation of enzymes is a much faster metabolic process than the synthesis of new proteins, peptide hormones act much more quickly than steroids and can fire up a metabolic pathway within minutes, while steroids take hours to exert their metabolic effect. Peptides are geared for rapid action, while steroids have a slower, more sustained impact on metabolic events.

Other Hormones

Several important hormones belong to neither the peptide nor the steroid group; rather they are small molecules synthesized from the precursor amino acid tyrosine. One such hormone, epinephrine, also known as adrenaline, has historically been of central importance to the field of endocrinology. The first hormone isolated in extracts and the first hormone to have its chemical structure determined, it was also used by Sutherland in his experiments on liver cells, which led to the discovery of cyclic AMP. Epinephrine is a life-preserving drug in the treatment of severe allergic reactions; in situations of severe stress it is released from the adrenal glands into the circulation to support lung and cardiovascular functions and to release metabolic fuels from storage sites.

Epinephrine is synthesized in the adrenal medulla cells from the amino acid tyrosine in a series of steps, each controlled by a specific enzyme. Two steps appear to be regulated by nerve impulses arriving from the sympathetic nervous system, and the final step, norepinephrine to epinephrine, is regulated by cortisol from the adrenal cortex. Epinephrine binds to receptors on the surface of its target cells and stimulates the formation of cyclic AMP as a second messenger, but it may also act via other second messengers. In general, then, epinephrine behaves like a peptide hormone, although it is very small and much different in structure from most peptides. It's the kind of hormone you like to have around when you are under attack from all directions by hostile creatures bent on unhinging you from your usual state of quiet repose.

Thyroxine, like epinephrine, is neither a peptide nor a steroid. Thyroid cells produce the two unique hormones called thyroxine (T4) and triiodothyronine (T3). These hormones contain four and three iodine atoms respectively; from these they derive their designation T4 and T3. The way T4 and T3 act on their target cells is unique. They diffuse directly into the cell cytoplasm, where T4 is converted to T3; the T3 then migrates into the cell nucleus to interact with a high-affinity protein receptor attached to DNA. This starts the production of messenger RNA, and the message calls for making certain specific proteins that the target cells need. T3 is the only hormone known to go directly into a target cell nucleus to operate without first binding to receptors in the plasma membrane or cytoplasm. It acts somewhat the way steroid hormones do in that it turns on mRNA synthesis inside the target cell nucleus.

Feedback Regulation

We now have formed a general view of hormone synthesis and action. These chemical messengers, which have evolved through eons of time from bacteria to humans, regulate vital processes throughout the body in a complex and yet somewhat coordinated fashion. Glands and other hormone-producing cell clusters respond to intimate chemical signals by the release of diverse peptides, steroids, and tyrosine derivatives into the circulation to seek out appropriate receptors at distant target cells. The resulting interactions are intertwined in such a way that there is method in the madness. Feedback signals from the target cells let the manufacturing glands know what is going on at the outskirts. Thyroxine from the thyroid signals the pituitary to back off with the TSH, just as cortisol does to adrenocorticotropic hormone (ACTH). A rising serum calcium level signals the parathyroid glands to ease up on the PTH production, and the synthesis of insulin by cells in the pancreas is constantly adjusted to hold the serum glucose level within acceptable bounds.

This intimacy between hormone synthesis and hormone action serves as the basis for a finely tuned network of chemical regulation whereby numerous biochemical processes throughout the body are coordinated. Over 3 billion years of natural selection to arrive at this fantastic scheme—with nature tinkering away, for better or worse, in the interest of survival until the design is streamlined into a unified whole. The hormones serve as a conduit of information, which allows the body to function at an optimal level and allows us to survive in the face of extraordinary changes in the surrounding environment.

3

ONE MILLION PIGS

■

The hypothalamus is the kind of place where one would expect plenty of intrigue. It is the Casablanca of the central nervous system—a place where mysterious messages from the brain are sorted out and scrambled into a new language of peptide hormones, a place where those of you who are inclined to the adventurous side of life would feel right at home. It has taken hundreds of investigators dozens of years of rummaging through the brains of over 1 million pigs and a similar number of sheep to identify the peptide hormones in the hypothalamus that regulate the pituitary gland. Never in the course of history have so many pigs contributed so much knowledge about so few hormones.

The *hypothalamus*, a small region of the brain located just above the pituitary gland, stands at the apex of the body's hormone network and is in charge of integrating signals coming from many regions of the nervous system. It is in the hypothalamus that nerve signals are first converted into hormone signals to begin a cascade to the pituitary and from there to the rest of the body. The discovery in the hypothalamus of hormones that regulate the pituitary gland has unfolded over the past several decades to become one of the most exciting chapters in the field of endocrine physiology. This discovery did not come easily; it required many frustrating years of effort in numerous laboratories throughout the world.

Because hypothalamic hormones are present in such minute quantities in the brain, their detection, isolation, and chemical identification is an extremely difficult undertaking. As, time after time, numerous investigators tried but failed to come up with the hormones, many

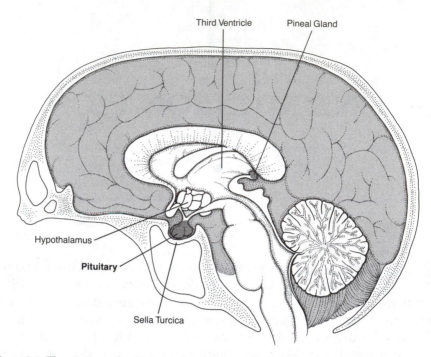

Third Ventricle   Pineal Gland

Hypothalamus

Pituitary

Sella Turcica

Figure 3-1. The pituitary gland is located at the base of the brain just beneath the hypothalamus within a bony structure called the sella turcica.

came to doubt that they even existed. Finally, after nearly 15 years of sustained effort, the laboratories of Schally and Guillemin—independently of each other—isolated the first hypothalamic hormone, TRH (thyrotropin-releasing hormone) in 1969, and determined its chemical structure. The starting material for Schally's isolation was the hypothalami from over 1 million pigs, and Guillemin required a similar number of sheep. To reach this milestone in neuroendocrine research was obviously not a task for the timid or the weak at heart. It was a feat of biomedical engineering on a monumental scale, requiring enormous resources in money and manpower, combined with will and determination.

Formation of a Theory

The *pituitary* is a small gland lying at the base of the brain in a bony cavity called the *sella turcica* (Turkish saddle). Known since antiquity, it was designated by the Greeks as the *hypophysis*, from *phyein*, meaning "to grow." Thus the pituitary or hypophysis is a growth below the brain and is connected to the brain by a short stalk (see Figure 3-1).

In the second century A.D. it was viewed by the renowned physician Galen as a dumping ground, where waste products from the brain accumulated after flowing down the pituitary stalk. From the pituitary the waste supposedly drained through the sinuses into the nose, where it appeared as *pituita* (nasal mucus), from which the name pituitary is derived. Surprisingly, this view persisted for 1,500 years—until the seventeenth century, when Schneider in Germany and Lower in England demonstrated experimentally that it was impossible under normal circumstances for fluid to pass from the brain to the nose. It was not until the twentieth century that the pituitary gland came to be viewed as a master gland that secretes numerous hormones into the bloodstream to regulate the body's physiology.

Detailed anatomical and physiological studies of the pituitary carried out in this century have revealed it to be an extraordinary organ regulating the hormone output of many other glands throughout the body. The anterior part, or *adenohypophysis*, secretes LH and FSH to control the gonads, TSH to control the thyroid gland, and ACTH to control the adrenal glands, as well as growth hormone and prolactin. The posterior part, or *neurohypophysis*, secretes vasopressin (also known as antidiuretic hormone or ADH) to regulate water metabolism, and oxytocin to control uterus contractions and breast milk ejection at the time of delivery. All of these hormones are peptides that were for a long time believed to be controlled by simple feedback regulation mechanisms. The twentieth century concept of the pituitary as a master gland in charge of regulating metabolic events throughout the body gradually came to encompass the notion that the pituitary itself was regulated by higher centers in the brain, such as the hypothalamus. The discovery that the pituitary hormones were released in response to many different stimuli from the environment could not be explained without invoking pathways between the nervous system and the pituitary gland.

How the posterior pituitary is regulated by the brain was the first problem to be solved (see Figure 3-2). As early as 1894 Ramón y Cajal discovered a tract of nerve fibers running from the hypothalamus to the posterior pituitary, and other investigators later verified that the posterior pituitary contains a rich supply of nerves originating in the regions of the hypothalamus. Located near the optic tract and the third ventricle of the brain, they are called the supraoptic and paraventricular nerve clusters. The posterior pituitary hormones (vasopressin and oxytocin) are synthesized in these hypothalamic nerve clusters and

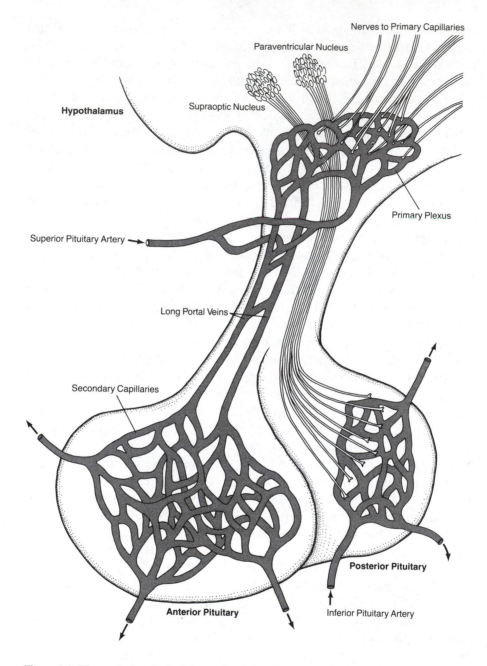

Figure 3-2. The posterior pituitary is regulated directly by nerve tracts from the paraventricular and supraoptic nerve clusters (called nuclei) in the hypothalamus. The anterior pituitary is regulated by hypothalamic hormones like TRH that are released into the portal circulation between the hypothalamus and the pituitary gland.

are then transported in granules down the nerve axons to the posterior pituitary, where they are stored in the nerve endings. Vasopressin and oxytocin are released from the posterior pituitary when appropriate stimuli from the bloodstream or from the nervous system reach the hypothalamus.

Here was an elegant demonstration that the brain and the *posterior* pituitary gland are connected by a set of unique nerve cells capable of synthesizing hormones to achieve a remarkable unification of the nervous system and the endocrine system. The release of vasopressin and oxytocin at the right time is controlled directly by nerve cells that originate in the hypothalamus and extend into the posterior pituitary. These hormones are made in the hypothalamus and stored in the nerve cells ending in the pituitary; when they are needed elsewhere in the body they are then secreted into the circulation.

To discern how the nervous system was integrated with the *anterior* pituitary was not so simple, and the search for the answer frustrated investigators for many years. In the first place, no nerve fibers from the hypothalamus or from anywhere else in the brain could be identified in the anterior pituitary. How then could signals be sent from the brain to the anterior pituitary to release hormones into the circulation? Certainly not by the simple type of neuron pathway seen in the posterior pituitary.

By the 1930s it was well known that in mammals the central nervous system exerts a precise control over the release of gonadotropins (LH and FSH) from the anterior pituitary, but no one knew how this was accomplished. It had been known since 1797 that female rabbits ovulate several hours after mating, and it was subsequently shown that this occurred because mating initiated reflex signals from the spinal cord to the brain, which caused the release of LH from the anterior pituitary. Ovulation, it was discovered, could be initiated by many other stimuli, such as temperature, light, food supply, and psychological factors. The hypothalamus became implicated in the final pathway between the brain and the pituitary when researchers, by inserting electric probes into various regions of the hypothalamus of rabbits, demonstrated that electrical stimulation of this region of the brain could induce ovulation in rabbits and other animals. Similar electrical stimulation of the hypothalamus could also cause the release of ACTH, TSH, and growth hormone from the pituitary, while direct stimulation of the pituitary gland caused no release of pituitary hormones.

Another finding confirmed the dependence of the pituitary upon stimulation from the hypothalamus: Destructive lesions in the hypothalamus caused a decrease in the secretion of pituitary hormones. So it was clear that the integrity of the hypothalamus is critical for the relay of information from the central nervous system to the pituitary. The hypothalamus was obviously the key link between the nervous system and the endocrine system, but the details of this linkage had to wait until the anatomical connections between the hypothalamus and the anterior pituitary were discovered. It was generally assumed that the two were connected by nerve fibers not yet identified.

A break came in the early 1930s when Popa and Fielding, through a series of detailed anatomical studies, found blood vessels (called the *hypothalamic-pituitary portal system*) connecting capillary vessels of the hypothalamus to capillary vessels of the pituitary; they incorrectly inferred, however, that blood flow was *to* the hypothalamus *from* the pituitary. Wislocki and King then showed that blood flowed *from* the hypothalamus down through the portal system in the pituitary stalk *to* the anterior pituitary gland. The stage was now set for a revolutionary new theory explaining how the pituitary was regulated by the hypothalamus, a theory that was the intellectual driving force for experiments in neuroendocrinology for the next 20 years.

This theory, put forward by Geoffrey Harris and several other investigators, suggested that nerve cells in the hypothalamus synthesize hormones that are released directly into the capillary blood vessels of the hypothalamus, from where they flow via the portal system to the pituitary gland. Here the hypothalamic hormones stimulate cells to release pituitary hormones directly into the general circulation (see Figure 3-2). The new theory accounted for the absence of nerve fibers connecting the hypothalamus to the anterior pituitary, as well as for the presence of a unique system of blood vessels in the pituitary stalk through which blood flowed from the hypothalamus to the pituitary. The same theory also postulated a mechanism by which nerve pathways in the central nervous system could lead to release of pituitary hormones, namely by stimulating nerve cells in the hypothalamus. Harris was not only the leading proponent of this theory but also provided much of the experimental foundation to support it. The Harris conjecture about hypothalamic-releasing hormones, showing how the brain could regulate the anterior pituitary gland and thereby control hormone secretion from important glands throughout the body, was of central importance in the field of endocrinology.

TABLE 3-1

Hormones Produced in the Hypothalamus

Hormone Designation	Name of Hypothalamic Hormone
CRH	Corticotropin-Releasing Hormone
GHRH	Growth-Hormone-Releasing Hormone
Somatostatin	Growth-Hormone-Release-Inhibiting Hormone
LHRH	Luteinizing-Hormone-Releasing Hormone
PIH	Prolactin-Inhibiting Hormone
PRH	Prolactin-Releasing Hormone
TRH	Thyrotropin-Releasing Hormone

The first line of evidence to support the new theory came from animal experiments in which the pituitary stalk was cut (or sectioned) to disconnect the hypothalamus from the pituitary gland, an experiment that was simple in concept but difficult to carry out. Harris showed that previous similar experiments often failed to prevent hormone release from the pituitary gland because the portal blood vessels avidly regenerated across the cut portion of the stalk. When, however, he inserted a plate across the cut to prevent portal blood vessel regeneration, the animals invariably failed to ovulate, proving that for the pituitary release of LH and FSH to occur these blood vessels had to be connected. Research by other investigators using different animals soon confirmed this work.

In his next experiments, Harris, working with Jacobsohn, removed the pituitary gland from its natural location in the sella turcica and transplanted it elsewhere in the brain, where it was revascularized by blood vessels not connected to the hypothalamus; in this experiment the pituitary gland failed to release gonadotropins and therefore ovulation did not occur. However, when the pituitary was transplanted near the hypothalamus, ovulation occurred and the animals became pregnant after mating. Further investigation by others showed that if the pituitary gland is transplanted to places in the body remote from the sella turcica, the pituitary hormones (ACTH, LH, FSH, TSH, and GH) are not secreted; but if the pituitary is put back where it belongs, beneath the hypothalamus, these hormones are released normally. These observations provided strong experimental evidence that the hypothalamus controls the pituitary gland via the portal circulation. It remained then to isolate and identify the hypothalamic hormones that regulate the pituitary gland (see Table 3-1).

The Initial Attack

The validity of this radically new theory of pituitary regulation hinged on the existence in the hypothalamus of unique hormones that could induce the release of pituitary hormones into the general circulation. A long and arduous struggle began in numerous laboratories to isolate the hypothetical hypothalamic-releasing hormones or releasing "factors" as they were designated initially during the early days, when their very existence was subject to considerable doubt.

The initial step in approaching the problem of isolating hypothalamic hormones was a demonstration that the hormones actually existed. The only reliable assay for a pituitary hormone available in the early 1950s was the assay for adrenocorticotropic hormone (ACTH), the peptide hormone that regulates the synthesis of cortisol in the adrenal glands. Since an assay was available, it was natural that the hypothalamic hormone that induced the release of ACTH from the pituitary—corticotropin-releasing hormone (CRH)—would be the first point of attack to prove the Harris theory.

As so often happens in scientific research, two groups of investigators working independently, without knowledge of each other's efforts, simultaneously hit upon firm evidence for the existence of CRH by very similar experiments. Guillemin and Rosenberg in Houston cultured anterior pituitary cells from rats and dogs in test tubes and showed, as others had before, that after several days the cells were no longer capable of making ACTH, which disappeared from the culture medium. This decline in production of ACTH occurred despite the fact that the pituitary cells remained metabolically viable and went right on growing. The critical part of the experiment was the addition of hypothalamic tissue to the culture of pituitary cells. As this tissue was added, the pituitary cells produced more and more ACTH—evidence that the cells from the hypothalamus contributed some factor that could stimulate the release of ACTH from pituitary cells. This factor behaved like the hypothesized CRH. At the same time, Saffran and Schally in Montreal, using rat anterior pituitary tissue, reached similar conclusions, shown schematically in Figure 3-3. The discoveries of these two groups were published in 1955 and prepared the way for a monumental experimental effort to isolate and identify CRH, an effort that was finally successful in 1981—26 years later. The central importance of corticotropin-releasing hormone lies not only in the fact that it controls ACTH and cortisol production, but also in its having

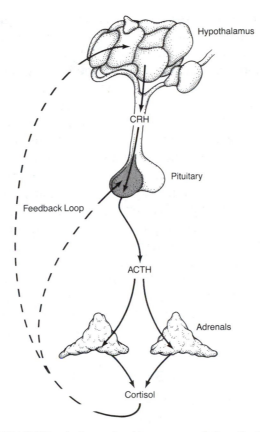

Figure 3-3. The CRH/ACTH/cortisol cascade of hormone regulation. Cortisol regulates its own synthesis by feedback suppression (dashed line) of CRH and ACTH synthesis.

been the first hypothalamic hormone whose isolation was attempted in a serious way.

Test tube cultures of pituitary cells could be used as an assay for CRH, but the amount of CRH present in the hypothalamus of a single animal was pitifully small, too small ever to allow the chemical determination of CRH. The hypothalami from a large number of animals had to be obtained. The goal was to gear up to an industrial scale and proceed with the identification of the chemical structure of CRH. Guillemin and Hearn began by obtaining beef hypothalami from a Houston meat packing house. They worked out a method to partially purify CRH by grinding up the hypothalamic cells and extracting the cell contents with special solvents. The components of the extract were then separated by a technique known as paper chromatography. Even so, they were unable to isolate enough material to attempt a determination of the structure of CRH. Other investigators were beginning to have doubts about the existence of CRH, arguing that the posterior pituitary hormone vasopressin (also known as ADH or antidiuretic hormone) could stimulate ACTH release from pituitary cells, and therefore vasopressin might interfere with the CRH assay.

The isolation of CRH posed enormous technical difficulties. In 1957 Schally left Montreal and joined Guillemin in Houston to work on this problem. These two tenacious investigators (who eventually shared the Nobel Prize for their research) made little progress on CRH. The hormone was elusive, and activity seemed to disappear from the extracts whenever further purification was attempted. Further chromatography techniques were employed but they were insufficient. The attempt to find CRH had intractable ambiguities, and so, after seven years of effort, the search for the structure of CRH was abandoned while the search for other hypothalamic hormones continued. Schally left Houston in 1962 to set up his own laboratory at the Veterans Administration Hospital in New Orleans. An epic race began between Schally and Guillemin to isolate and identify the first hypothalamic hormone.

The Race for TRH

Guillemin had moved to Paris in 1960 to set up a laboratory at the Collège de France while still maintaining his research group in Houston, where Schally was still grinding away on the ill-fated CRH isolation project. In Paris Guillemin changed course and decided to try to isolate the hypothalamic-releasing hormones LHRH (luteinizing-hormone-releasing hormone) and TRH (thyrotropin-releasing hormone). The isolation of a releasing hormone in a pure form was essential in order to proceed with the determination of its chemical structure. He processed over five tons of hypothalamic tissue from 500,000 sheep in Paris, and with the development of an accurate assay for the detection of TRH made considerable progress in the isolation of TRH. But Guillemin had a falling out with his colleagues in Paris and returned to Houston in 1963, shortly after Schally had left for New Orleans to set up a rival laboratory. In Houston, Guillemin organized a new research group, which included Vale and the chemist Burgus. This new group continued the work begun in Paris, for which they now processed the hypothalami of nearly 2 million sheep into extracts for a frontal assault on the structure of TRH. Here was a chemical engineer's dream world, where large vats of material could be sloshed around to produce extracts that would be purified on industrial-scale chromatography columns. This bold adventure required large sums of money from the National Institutes of Health and an enormous amount of scientific effort—certainly there was no place here for a timid approach to the problem. The effort began to show results; in 1964 the Guillemin group reported that TRH contained 11 amino acids, and by 1965 they had upgraded this estimate to 18 amino acids.

Schally was not standing idly by while all this was going on. He had been recruited to New Orleans in late 1962 by Bowers, an endocrinologist at Tulane University School of Medicine. Shortly after arriving in New Orleans, Schally set up his own research group at the Veterans Administration Hospital. Like Guillemin, he abandoned the pursuit of CRH and eventually focused his attention on TRH. At this point he was well behind Guillemin in the isolation of this hypothalamic hormone; he therefore decided to use pig hypothalami as a source of extracts because Guillemin was using sheep hypothalami. If Guillemin determined the chemical structure of sheep TRH first, then Schally would still have important publishable results even if pig TRH turned out to be identical in structure to sheep TRH.

Schally needed a source of pig hypothalami that would not be too expensive for his modest research budget, and he hit upon a bonanza. The meat packer Oscar Mayer in Wisconsin slaughtered 10,000 pigs a day; the company generously agreed to give Schally the hypothalami from these pigs in lots of 100,000. Over time the Oscar Mayer Company donated more than 1 million pig hypothalami to Schally's laboratory, a gift that was crucial to his research effort. Through intense effort expended on the purification of pig hypothalamus extracts, Schally's group made considerable progress in the purification of TRH; they reported in early 1966 that pig TRH contained up to 23 amino acids.

It was at this juncture that both the Schally and Guillemin research groups swerved sharply in the wrong direction, a blunder that was nearly fatal to their investigative efforts. The Guillemin group, after concluding that TRH was composed of 18 amino acids, embarked on a massive experiment to determine its exact structure. They processed another five tons of hypothalamic tissue from 500,000 sheep through several solvent extractions followed by a series of separate purification steps. They determined that TRH contained only 5 to 8 percent amino acids by weight and concluded, therefore, in May 1966, that TRH was not a simple peptide composed only of amino acids. The experiment yielded incorrect results, probably as a result of contamination during the purification steps.

Schally's group, not to be outdone, processed 100,000 pig hypothalami through a number of meticulous purification steps and surprisingly came up with the right answer: that TRH was composed of only three amino acids—*histidine, glutamic acid*, and *proline*. However, they miscalculated the purity of their final sample and concluded that these amino acids accounted for only 30 percent of the weight of TRH. This led them to the same false hypothesis as Guillemin—that TRH was not a simple peptide consisting only of amino acids. Schally even had the Merck Sharp and Dohme pharmaceutical company synthesize all six tripeptides, representing all of the possible permutations of the three amino acids—histidine, glutamic acid, and proline (see Figure 3-4). None of these showed any TRH biological activity. The identity of TRH remained hidden from view.

glu-his-pro	glu-pro-his
his-glu-pro	his-pro-glu
pro-his-glu	pro-glu-his

Figure 3-4. The six possible tripeptide combinations of the amino acids glutamic acid (glu), histidine (his), and proline (pro). Only the glu-his-pro tripeptide could be converted to a molecule with TRH activity.

Schally and Guillemin had independently painted themselves into the same corner; they had reached an impasse based on the erroneous conclusion that TRH was not a simple peptide. This conclusion was not widely accepted in the scientific community; those who continued to believe that hypothalamic-regulating hormones existed still favored the view that they were most likely peptides, since the two posterior pituitary hormones, vasopressin and oxytocin, had both been proven to be simple peptides, each composed of nine amino acids. The relationship between Schally and Guillemin began to deteriorate and their rivalry began to show unusual antagonism at scientific meetings and in publications. This was not the ordinary type of academic squabble, where the infighting is so often vicious because the issues are so small;

rather the issues were important and the stakes were high. The investigator who isolated one of these hypothalamic hormones and determined its chemical structure would acquire a considerable amount of personal satisfaction, fame, and fortune in the form of research grants and prize money.

The Schally group abandoned their pursuit of TRH even though they had come exceedingly close to identifying its correct structure in late 1966. Instead they chose to work on other hypothalamic hormones, LHRH and GHRH (growth-hormone-releasing hormone). In 1968 Schally's NIH research funds were slashed by 40 percent, a warning that after seven years of unsuccessful effort to isolate CRH and another six years of going nowhere with TRH, the NIH in particular and the scientific community in general were losing patience with his futile efforts. An NIH-sponsored conference was arranged for January 1969, in Tucson, Arizona, to review the work of Guillemin and Schally, both of whom were perilously close to having their NIH research funding terminated. The leading investigators in the field of neuroendocrine research, including Geoffrey Harris, were brought together from around the world to pass judgment on the lack of progress in the isolation of hypothalamic hormones.

After the disastrous turn of events, when both Guillemin and Schally had concluded that TRH was not a simple peptide, Burgus in Guillemin's laboratory continued to work diligently behind the scenes to further purify TRH from sheep hypothalamic extracts. By the time of the Tucson conference he had, in fact, made considerable progress. At the conference Burgus made the dramatic announcement that TRH was composed of at least 80 percent amino acids and that the only detectable amino acids in TRH were glutamic acid, histidine, and proline, the same amino acids that Schally had identified in 1966. This was an important advance, and implied that the structure of TRH was within reach. It also assured the continuation of NIH funding in the nick of time.

Capitalizing on the fact that three different objects can be arranged in a linear sequence in six different ways, the Guillemin group had the six tripeptides that can be formed from glutamic acid, histidine, and proline synthesized by Hoffman La Roche in Switzerland, and discovered, as Schally had with Merck's same tripeptides three years earlier, that none of the six tripeptides had any TRH activity. Thus the structure of TRH remained a mystery even though the composition seemed fairly certain.

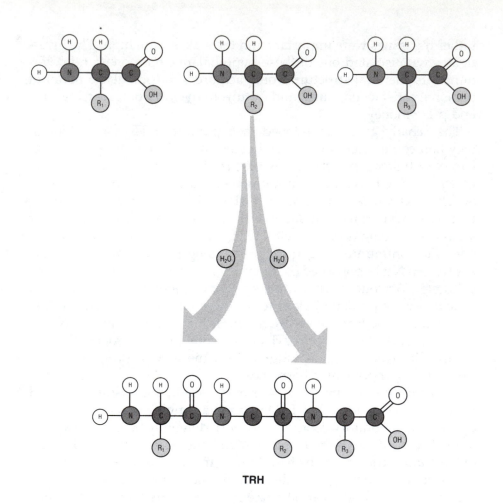

TRH

Figure 3-5. Three amino acids link together by peptide bonds to form a tripeptide chain. Some polypeptides and proteins are composed of many amino acids linked together by peptide bonds.

It was at this juncture in early 1969 that Burgus made a key break-through in the mystery of TRH, a breakthrough that hinged on his knowledge of peptide chemistry as well as some good fortune. When amino acids link together to form a peptide molecule (see Figure 3-5), there is a characteristically free amino acid group (NH_2) at one end and a free carboxyl group (COOH) at the other end, designated as the N-terminal and C-terminal ends of the peptide molecule. Burgus verified a previous Schally finding that TRH contains no free N-terminal; that is, the amino acid group at one end of TRH was blocked by bonding to some other chemical constituent.

The problem was to find out what caused this blockade. Since several natural peptides were known to be blocked at the N-terminal end by an acetyl group, Burgus decided to acetylate the N-terminal of all six tripeptide combinations of glutamic acid (glu), histidine (his), and proline (pro), the three amino acids in TRH (see Figure 3-4). To his surprise, only the acetylated tripeptide arranged in the order glu-his-pro showed TRH biological activity when assayed in animals, while none of the other acetylated tripeptides showed any TRH activity. The Guillemin group published this result in April 1969.

They soon discovered that the TRH activity resulting from the acetylation reaction of glu-his-pro was inadvertently produced by an unintended byproduct, pyro-glu-his-pro. Since this interesting molecule was not as active as their TRH extract in the animal assay, they synthesized several derivatives, including pyro-glu-his-pro-amide (see Figure 3-6), which they concluded was very similar to TRH but was not TRH itself. The Guillemin group was now on the verge of determining the structure of TRH, while the Schally group had thus far revealed nothing in print about their efforts to characterize TRH. After several more months of intense work, the Guillemin group finally

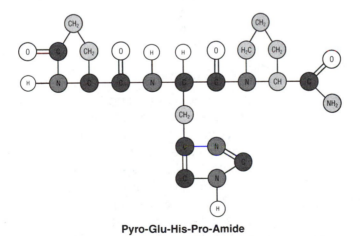

Pyro-Glu-His-Pro-Amide

Figure 3-6. It took two research groups seven years to show that TRH is pyro-glu-his-pro-amide, the first hypothalamic releasing hormone to be isolated and characterized chemically.

concluded that TRH was pyro-glu-his-pro-amide and submitted their exciting result for publication.

While they were celebrating and awaiting the November 12 publication of their momentous discovery, the bombshell exploded. On November 6, the Schally group published the structure of TRH—pyro-glu-his-pro-amide. After seven years of effort, Schally had won the race for TRH by a mere week, a reality that to this day Guillemin has still not accepted. However, by any fair analysis the race for TRH would be declared a dead heat.

How had Schally managed to catch up with Guillemin after appearing so hopelessly behind? Shortly after the Tucson conference in January 1969, where Burgus had announced the progress of the Guillemin group in the isolation and purification of TRH, Schally recruited the eminent chemist Folkers and his postdoctoral student Enzmann to help in a new concerted attack on the TRH problem, realizing that time was running out and an infusion of new talent into the effort was necessary. This maneuver paid off. By the end of February, Enzmann had confirmed that the amino acid sequence of TRH was glu-his-pro and that both the N-terminal and C-terminal ends were blocked. In May, Enzmann stumbled onto the sequence pyro-glu-his-pro-amide by an unintended side reaction, and over the next several months the Schally group was able to demonstrate that this sequence was identical to TRH. With the publication of this discovery in November 1969, one week before Guillemin's group published the same result, Harris's theory of hypothalamic-releasing hormones was validated and a new era of neuroendocrinology was begun.

The Second Race

The dust had hardly settled on TRH when Schally and Guillemin entered the race for LHRH (luteinizing-hormone-releasing hormone), an exceedingly important hypothalamic hormone that regulates reproductive capabilities and secondary sexual characteristics in women and men. LHRH acts directly on the pituitary to release LH (luteinizing hormone) and FSH (follicle-stimulating hormone) that travel through the bloodstream to the gonads (see Figure 3-7). The structure of LHRH was obviously of major interest to many scientists and pharmaceutical companies because of the central role of LHRH in regulating reproduction, with important implications for male and female contraception. Schally and Guillemin had competition in this race—very talented competition already well out ahead of them in determining the struc-

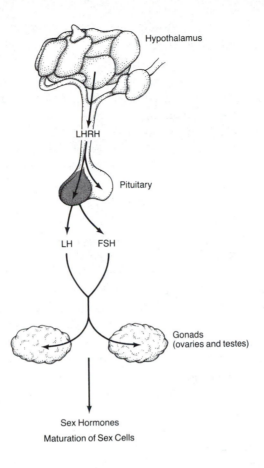

Hypothalamus

LHRH

Pituitary

LH   FSH

Gonads
(ovaries and testes)

Sex Hormones
Maturation of Sex Cells

Figure 3-7. LHRH stimulates the release of luteinizing hormone (LH) and follicle-stimulating hormone (FSH) from the anterior pituitary gland. LH and FSH regulate the reproductive glands.

ture of LHRH—from two scientists, Harris and McCann, both of whom had a long-standing interest in the structure of LHRH. In 1960 each had independently reported experimental evidence for the existence of LHRH; by late 1969, while Schally and Guillemin were still locked in their struggle to determine the structure of TRH, Mc-Cann and Harris were independently closing in on the structure of LHRH.

McCann was born and raised in Texas, and in 1965 he established at the University of Texas in Dallas one of the world's leading laboratories in neuroendocrinology. By 1969 he and his chemist Fawcett had obtained a highly purified sample of LHRH to use for chemical analysis. A year later they reported that LHRH was a small peptide, blocked at both ends like TRH.

Harris in England was also getting warm. By May 1970, he and his chemist Gregory had isolated nearly pure LHRH and shown that it contained from 9 to 13 amino acids. It was Harris, you will remember, who had formulated the theory of hypothalamic regulation and thus provided the intellectual foundation for all of the isolation work. The theory had been validated by the purification and identification of TRH, and now he was within reach of identifying LHRH. However, both Harris and McCann failed in their quest for LHRH for similar reasons. They were both academic physiologists with broad interests in the physiology of pituitary regulation; neither of them was willing to commit all of his resources to isolation work and to set aside the more intellectually stimulating physiology. Even so, each came remarkably close to establishing the structure of LHRH.

Finally, the race for LHRH, as for TRH, boiled down to a struggle between the laboratories of Schally and Guillemin, both of whom were totally committed to isolation work. While Harris and McCann were working with thousands of animal hypothalami, Schally and Guillemin were working with millions; it was a difference of pounds versus tons of tissue, flasks versus vats of extract, and nanograms versus micrograms of hormone. To play successfully in this league, you had to gear up to an industrial scale and then commit yourself to an around-the-clock effort.

In June 1970 Guillemin moved his laboratory from the Baylor College of Medicine in Houston to the Salk Institute in La Jolla, California, which cost him precious time in the LHRH race. Burgus used all of their carefully preserved TRH extracts as a starting point and by the end of the year he had made considerable progress in the purification of LHRH. He determined that LHRH contained nine amino acids and was blocked on one end by pyro-glutamate and on the other end by an amide group similar to TRH. But Guillemin and Burgus had only about 40 micrograms of LHRH (a barely visible quantity), not enough to perform an amino acid sequencing experiment. They had to procure another 500,000 sheep hypothalami and go through the whole series of steps necessary to obtain a larger quantity of purified LHRH.

During the same year Schally's group processed 160,000 pig hypothalami to obtain approximately 250 micrograms of LHRH—over five times the amount Guillemin's group had. By January 1971 they too concluded that LHRH contained nine amino acids and was blocked on both ends. They further estimated that even 250 micrograms of LHRH was not enough to determine its structure. Schally therefore recruited the talented Japanese chemist Matsuo to New Orleans. Schally was assisted in this recruitment by his Japanese co-worker, Arimura, who had already recruited Baba from Tokyo to help with the structural analysis of LHRH. Matsuo wasted no time and immediately infused the project with new momentum by an ingenious experiment. In collaboration with Baba he quickly determined that LHRH was composed of ten amino acids, not nine amino acids as Guillemin and Schally had both previously concluded. Matsuo made this discovery using only five micrograms of the 250 microgram LHRH stock, but the remaining material was too small to determine the amino acid sequence of LHRH by a conventional approach.

Matsuo then convinced Schally to hold off on the announcement of the ten-amino-acid structure of LHRH while he went to work on the detailed analysis. By this maneuver they risked losing priority in the discovery of ten amino acids, but they gained by not revealing what they knew and thereby bought some time to sequence LHRH. Because of the small amount of LHRH available, Matsuo had to take some daring chemical shortcuts; this paid big dividends, for he soon arrived at a structure close to LHRH, with only one amino acid position left to determine. Finally, he synthesized a peptide candidate for LHRH by guessing where the final amino acid would go, and in late April 1971, Arimura tested Matsuo's synthetic product in a new radioimmunoassay and showed that it was in fact LHRH. In less than four months after his arrival at Schally's lab from Japan, Matsuo had accomplished a task of chemical analysis that was widely considered impossible at that time, and he had used only 50 micrograms of Schally's precious 250 microgram LHRH stock.

The result of this second monumental breakthrough in hypothalamic neurochemistry was announced to the world by Schally at the Endocrine Society meeting in San Francisco on June 24, 1971, and was published shortly thereafter. LHRH is a decapeptide (it contains ten amino acids) which, like TRH, has a pyroglutamate group at one end and an amide group at the other. This important molecule stimulates both LH and FSH release from the pituitary, implying that LHRH is the hypothalamic-releasing hormone for FSH as well as LH. In fact, to date no one has yet discovered an independent follicle-stimulating-hormone-releasing hormone in the hypothalamus of animals or humans.

Schally's team had won the race for LHRH by a wide margin compared to his victory in the TRH race, and against formidable opposition that included Guillemin, Harris, and McCann, whose research programs on the structural determination of LHRH were devastated by the Schally announcement. Just as Folkers and Enzmann had provided a critical thrust for Schally in determining the chemical structure of TRH, the Japanese chemists Matsuo and Baba, along with their countryman Arimura, had done the same for LHRH. Time was running out on Schally, however, and the winds of fortune were about to blow in a new direction.

The Third Hypothalamic Hormone

With the structure of TRH and LHRH known and the Harris theory of hypothalamic-pituitary regulation on sound scientific footing, attention turned toward the regulation of growth hormone. The Harris theory proposed that there was one hypothalamic-releasing hormone for each anterior pituitary hormone and that a growth-hormone-releasing hormone (GHRH) should therefore exist. When evidence for the existence of such a factor had been published by Deuben and Meites several years earlier, Schally had begun his attempt to isolate GHRH. By 1971, after five years of effort, Schally and his co-workers had purified a 10-amino-acid molecule that had the properties of GHRH in one assay but not in the other tests. They determined the structure of this putative GHRH and published the result in a prestigious scientific journal. Unfortunately, they made a major error in the isolation steps and came up with a fragment of pig hemoglobin that just happened to assay like GHRH in the one assay Schally had decided to use for the isolation. It was a bitter lesson—large scale isolations involving tons of tissue easily give rise to impurities that can mimic the desired product.

In the meantime Guillemin's fortunes took a turn for the better by a serendipitous route. He too was attempting to isolate GHRH and had assigned the task to a young Canadian student named Brazeau, who had just joined the Guillemin research group. Brazeau, using a new sensitive assay system for GHRH developed by Vale in cultures of pituitary cells from rats, soon discovered that hypothalamic extracts inhibit the release of growth hormone from the pituitary (he mercifully designated this inhibitor as somatostatin, because growth hormone is also known as somatotropin) in 1968. Burgus, in Guillemin's laboratory, proceeded rapidly with the isolation of somatostatin and determined its chemical sequence, which he published in January 1973. Somatostatin is a 14-amino-acid polypeptide with the remarkable property that at very low concentrations it inhibits growth hormone secretion from the pituitary gland. To date it is the only hypothalamic hormone to be elucidated that inhibits the secretion of a pituitary hormone, although such a hypothalamic hormone is postulated to exist for the pituitary hormone prolactin. Interestingly, somatostatin has recently been shown to be present in the gut and in the pancreas gland, where it inhibits the release of insulin and glucagon. Thus, wherever it is found in the body, somatostatin seems to suppress the release of neighboring hormones.

With the isolation of TRH, LHRH, and somatostatin the curtain came down on the first phase of the identification of hypothalamic hormones and verification of the hormonal theory of pituitary regulation by the brain via the hypothalamus. All three of these important hormones have been used in medical research, diagnostic testing, or therapy.

The Return to CRH

The Harris theory of hypothalamic regulation had nearly foundered on the rocks of the initial failed attempt to isolate corticotropin-releasing hormone (CRH). Guillemin and Schally had discovered the existence of CRH as a stimulator of ACTH release from pituitary cells in 1955 and then spent the next seven years in a futile effort to isolate and purify it. The problem was too tough; it was the Everest of hormone isolations—the initial assays for CRH were primitive and lacked accuracy, CRH was very unstable, and other hormones (such as vasopressin) seemed to get in the way of the purification. For these reasons CRH was placed on the back burner while the easier isolations of TRH, LHRH, and somatostatin unfolded. A breakthrough was needed that would allow research on the structure of CRH to move forward.

The breakthrough came in the early and mid-1970s, when an assay for CRH was perfected. The assay employed cells isolated from rat pituitary glands and a very sensitive radioimmunoassay for ACTH so that small quantities of CRH, the hormone that stimulates the pituitary cells to make ACTH in a test tube could be detected. Finally, after years of work, Vale and his colleagues at the Salk Institute in La Jolla reported the structure of CRH in September 1981; it was the largest hypothalamic hormone reported to date—41 amino acids long. The CRH hormone was found in the hypothalamic extracts from 490,000 sheep which had been used for the LHRH isolation and had been meticulously saved for future research. It was quickly shown that the newly discovered CRH stimulates ACTH release from the pituitary gland of humans and other animals, apparently by stimulating the release of cyclic AMP inside the ACTH-secreting cells. The discovery of the structure of CRH in 1981 brought to a close a frustrating chapter of 25 years of research begun in 1955—and opened up a whole new line of investigation on the mechanism of action of CRH and its location in the brain.

The Regulation of Growth Hormone

The existence in the hypothalamus of a hormone that regulates growth hormone release from the pituitary was first discovered in 1964, when extracts from the hypothalami of rats were shown by Deuben and Meites to stimulate growth hormone production in cultured rat anterior pituitary cells. After Schally had erroneously identified a fragment of pig hemoglobin as GHRH, it was back to the starting blocks with GHRH. During the 1970s several reports appeared proposing peptide structures with GHRH activity, but none of these structures showed high potency and all were discarded. The solution to this problem came from an unexpected direction.

Several adult patients who were suffering from an excess of growth hormone production were found to have a tumor in the pancreas gland. The pancreatic tumors were producing a substance that stimulated the pituitary gland to make too much growth hormone—that is, they were producing a growth-hormone-releasing factor that circulated to the pituitary.

In 1982 the two independent research laboratories of Guillemin and Vale, within six weeks of each other, submitted for publication articles demonstrating the structure of growth-hormone-releasing factor isolated from these human pancreas tumors (designated hpGRF, human pancreas growth-hormone-releasing factor). In the first case, two pancreatic tumors were removed from a young male patient with acromegaly in Lyon, France, and sent to Guillemin at the Salk Institute in La Jolla for analysis. Extracts of the tumor tissue yielded a 44-amino-acid hpGRF as well as several shorter fragments of this molecule—fragments of 40 and 37 amino acids with full biological activity.

Vale's group received pancreatic tumor tissue that had been removed from a 21-year-old acromegalic woman in Virginia from which they were able to isolate a single 40-amino-acid peptide hpGRF identical in

TABLE 3-2

Hypothalamic Hormone	Year Structure Discovered	Year Existence Discovered	Number of Peptide Amino Acids	Pituitary Action
TRH	1969	1961	3	TSH Release
LHRH	1971	1960	10	LH and FSH Release
Somatostatin	1973	1968	14	Growth Hormone Suppression
CRH	1981	1955	41	ACTH Release
GHRH	1982	1964	40	Growth Hormone Release
PRH	—	1960	—	Prolactin Release
PIH	—	1961	—	Prolactin Inhibitor

Characteristics of the Hypothalamic Hormones

sequence to Guillemin's 40-amino-acid hpGRF. Both research groups synthesized hpGRF from the component amino acids and showed that the molecule stimulates growth hormone release from the pituitaries of animals and humans.

The isolation of growth-hormone-releasing hormone (GHRH) from hypothalamic extracts has thus far not been accomplished, but there is good reason to believe that GHRH will turn out to be very similar if not identical in structure to hpGRF, since the latter peptide exhibits the exact physiological responses one would expect for GHRH.

The structures of all the hypothalamic regulatory hormones have now been discovered except for the hormones that regulate prolactin synthesis and release. The Harris theory of hypothalamic regulation of the pituitary gland has been fully validated with the isolation and identification thus far of five hypothalamic regulatory hormones (Table 3-2). Initially, proofs of the existence of these hormones were necessary to indicate that large-scale isolation experiments could succeed. These proofs took the form of experiments in which hypothalamic tissue or extracts could be shown to stimulate or inhibit the release of pituitary hormones from pituitary cells in culture. Often nearly a decade elapsed between an existence proof and the final identification of the structure of a hypothalamic regulatory hormone; in the case of CRH over 25 years elapsed. In the interim, a vigorous competition occurred between various research labs, involving many investigators and tons of tissue. In most instances, the people who developed the intellectual framework for hypothalamic regulation and who were involved in the existence proofs were not the same people who were successful in determining the structure of a given hormone—suggesting that a different approach and framework were needed for these different endeavors.

Validation of the Harris theory of regulation of the pituitary by hormones made in hypothalamic neurons has pushed the question about brain regulation of the pituitary back another step. The question now has become: How does the *brain* regulate the hypothalamic neurons that secrete the pituitary-regulating hormones?

4

THE MASTER GLAND

■

During the first half of the twentieth century, the endocrine system gradually came to be viewed as an orchestra in which the individual glands acted in concert to regulate essential metabolic processes. If a single component went astray—like a wrong note from the trumpet section—then the whole performance deteriorated; the body angled toward a state of ill health and remained out of tune until the problem was corrected. The conductor of this orchestra was perceived to be the pituitary gland, the master gland that guides the individual components in a fashion that produces harmony and efficient body function. Thus the pituitary was raised in conception from a repository of brain waste in antiquity to a master gland in the twentieth century!

In reality the pituitary is neither. (If there exists a master gland it is the brain, where multiple signals are received and then integrated into the hypothalamus, which in turn manufactures chemical messengers that regulate the pituitary.) Even though the pituitary gland is not today perceived as the ultimate regulator of the endocrine system, its clinical importance and intimate involvement in the regulation of numerous hormone systems is beyond dispute. It receives chemical signals from the brain via the hypothalamus and produces chemical messengers that enable it to regulate many different physiological processes throughout the body.

Ancient Views

The pituitary gland, buried deep in the brain below the third ventricle and hypothalamus (see Figure 3-1) hangs like an appendage at the base of the brain, inaccessible but known to anatomists for the past 2,000 years. Nothing about the location of the pituitary gland gives any clues to its vital importance in the regulation of the major hormone-producing glands. Its role remained an enigma surrounded by a cloud of conjecture and mythology until the twentieth century, when an explosion of hormone assays and well-designed experiments sorted the situation out.

The pituitary entered the twentieth century as a gland of ill repute, perceived as having little importance in the functioning of the body. There had been minimal headway during the eighteenth and nineteenth centuries, both in thinking and in experimental research related to the pituitary. Some interesting clues were unfolding during this time, however, suggesting that the pituitary might actually fill an important function. The embryonic origin of the anterior pituitary gland was demonstrated (by Rathke in 1838) to be the roof of the mouth—in contrast to the posterior pituitary, which originated from neural tissue of the brain. Since the anterior pituitary gland did not originate from the brain, there was no reason to expect it to transmit nerve signals in the usual way.

The first major insight into the function of the pituitary came from an unusual case. At age 24 a young woman had stopped menstruating. Her hands and feet began to enlarge, so that over the ensuing decade her shoe size increased markedly. She developed severe headaches and her jaw began to protrude forward. Her facial features thickened to an extent that made her barely recognizable to her family. The distinguished French neurologist Pierre Marie first described this patient in 1886—it was he who named the disorder acromegaly—but her complex disorder did not initiate a revolution in thinking about the pituitary gland. The chemical structure of human growth hormone was not finally determined until 1971, after nearly 100 years of investigation had unraveled many of the puzzling features of growth regulation by the pituitary gland.

Imagine what it would be like to wake up one morning and after fumbling your way through your usual up-and-at-'em rituals to notice that your shoes don't fit any more. Over the next several years you find yourself buying progressively larger shoes and cutting rings off your progressively enlarging fingers and hands. Then your jaw begins to protrude forward and the dental floss no longer gets stuck between your teeth. Your nose and lips begin to thicken and your forehead begins to furrow; doctors start peering at you in public places wondering if they should tell you what they think you've got. Throw in some headaches, some excessive sweating, a touch of impotence or amenorrhea and you've got yourself a full-blown case of acromegaly.

Several years later Marie noted that acromegaly was often associated with an enlargement of the pituitary gland arising from a pituitary tumor. He then reviewed the literature and found other similar cases, also with an enlarged pituitary, going back to the eighteenth century. Unfortunately, he wrongly concluded that the pituitary tumor was itself nonfunctional, that it merely interfered with the presumed growth-inhibiting role of the pituitary gland. The first person to suggest that the pituitary tumor itself produced something that stimulated growth in acromegaly was Minkowski; but this notion was not fashionable, and so the idea persisted that acromegaly resulted from damage to the anterior lobe of the pituitary gland.

With the advent of Schaefer's theory of internal secretions in 1895 and Starling's concept of hormones in 1905, thinking about the pituitary gland began to broaden. During the first decade of the twentieth century several critical observations and experiments were made. Fröhlich in Austria reported a new syndrome, in which obesity and lack of sexual development occurred in a young boy with a pituitary tumor, and other cases were soon reported. Paulesco in Rumania developed a surgical approach and showed that in dogs removal of the pituitary gland led to eventual death. Cushing, the famous Boston neurosurgeon, confirmed these experiments and then demonstrated that partial removal of the pituitary led to increased obesity, decreased sexual activity, and atrophy of the gonads; these events occurred only when the anterior pituitary was removed. Aschner provided convincing proof that removal of the pituitary also led to cessation of bone growth in young dogs.

So the idea unfolded that the pituitary is a ductless gland, secreting into the blood hormones that regulate growth and sexual development. As the century progressed, it was recognized that the anterior pituitary also regulates the thyroid, the adrenal glands, and milk production by the breasts. The pituitary came to be viewed as two distinct glands—an *anterior* gland regulating other glands throughout the body, and a *posterior* gland regulating water conservation and uterine contractions in women.

The Posterior Pituitary

Diabetes insipidus is actually quite an unusual disorder. Suddenly one day urine is pouring out like the Zambezi River hurling itself over

Victoria Falls, without any clear explanations—unceasing urination every 30 minutes or so with an unquenchable thirst in its wake. Diabetes is the Greek word for "siphon" and that is just what happens when the posterior pituitary gland or its nerve tracts from the hypothalamus are injured—water is siphoned from the body because the key hormone, vasopressin (also known as antidiuretic hormone [ADH] for obvious reasons) is missing. When ADH is missing, water cannot be retained in the body by the kidneys but leaks out at a furious pace. When this form of diabetes was first discovered, in 1794, the designation diabetes insipidus was used to distinguish the disorder from *diabetes mellitus*, in which sugar appears in the urine.

Although diabetes insipidus was well described in the medical literature thoughout the nineteenth century, it was not until 1912 that a connection between the pituitary gland and water conservation by the kidney was made. At that time a remarkable case was reported: A man who was shot in the head developed diabetes insipidus. What made the case remarkable was not simply that the patient survived to experience the increased frequency of urination, but that the bullet lodged in the sella turcica, where the pituitary gland is housed. Subsequent research demonstrated that lesions in specific regions of the hypothalamus and upper pituitary stalk in animals would produce diabetes insipidus. Pituitary extracts were shown to contain a substance that makes the kidneys conserve water (and is therefore an effective treatment for diabetes insipidus).

Neuroanatomists showed that the posterior gland is composed primarily of nerve fibers originating in the hypothalamus (see Figure 3-2). It remained to be discovered just exactly what it *did*; physiologists therefore started to make extracts from the posterior pituitary, which in many animals could be conveniently separated from the anterior pituitary. In 1898 Howell prepared some posterior pituitary extracts from sheep and injected the extract intravenously into dogs. The dogs' blood pressure increased. Between 1906 and 1913 a number of investigators showed that posterior pituitary extracts also stimulated uterus contractions, caused milk ejection from the breast, and had a water-conserving (antidiuretic) effect on the kidney. The researchers began to realize that all of these effects were caused by just two hormones, vasopressin and oxytocin.

Several more decades of work eventually led in the early 1950s to the isolation and synthesis of vasopressin and oxytocin—two small peptides, each composed of nine amino acids. These were the first

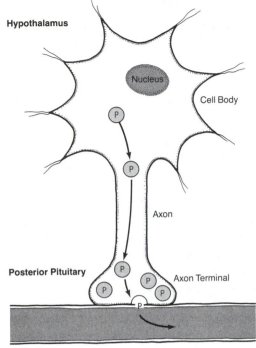

Figure 4-1. The peptides (P) vasopressin and oxytocin are synthesized in the bodies of nerve cells located in the hypothalamus and are then packaged into granules and transported down the nerve axon to be stored in the axon terminal until they are released into the circulation.

pituitary hormones to be characterized and then chemically synthesized. As understanding of posterior pituitary physiology increased, clinical use of the hormones became possible—vasopressin and its analogs for the treatment of diabetes insipidus, and oxytocin in obstetrics for the induction of labor (the name *oxytocin* stems from the Greek root meaning "quick birth").

Vasopressin and oxytocin are synthesized inside nerve cells located in specific regions of the hypothalamus. The hormones are packaged into granules and transported down the nerve cell axons into the posterior pituitary, where they are stored in the axon terminals (see Figure 4-1). One of the interesting features of this process is that vasopressin and oxytocin originate from similar precursor molecules, which are degraded by enzymes into both the hormones and carrier proteins called neurophysins. These carrier proteins are packaged in granules with the hormones so that neurophysin I accompanies vasopressin and neurophysin II is associated with oxytocin. The neu-

TABLE 4-1

Pituitary Hormones in Order of Size

Pituitary Hormone	Abbreviation	Amino Acids	Molecular Weight
Adrenocorticotropic Hormone	ACTH	39	4,500
Growth Hormone	GH	191	21,800
Prolactin	PRL	198	22,500
Luteinizing Hormone	LH	204	29,000
Follicle-Stimulating Hormone	FSH	204	29,000
Thyroid-Stimulating Hormone	TSH	204	29,000

rophysins apparently play a protective role and are released into the circulation along with their hormones when the nerve cells are triggered by stimuli reaching the hypothalamus. Vasopressin is released whenever the body needs to conserve water, and oxytocin is released to stimulate contractions of the uterus during childbirth. It's nice to have some vasopressin around whenever you are going for a long stroll on a hot day. It's nice to have some oxytocin around when you are trying to deliver a baby.

To summarize, the posterior pituitary is composed of nerve axons and nerve terminals that originate in the hypothalamus; these receive, from elsewhere in the brain, nerve signals concerning the conservation of water or childbirth and nurturing. These posterior pituitary neurons are neurosecretory cells that synthesize two hormones, vasopressin and oxytocin. God alone knows why these two hormones, so different in function, are so similar in structure and are so intimately associated in the pituitary.

The Anterior Pituitary

The anterior region of the pituitary is completely unrelated to the posterior pituitary in its embryological origin, in its regulatory function, and in its regulation by the hypothalamus. It took a long time to discover that the anterior pituitary secretes six important hormones (see Table 4-1). The discovery and characterization of the six anterior pituitary hormones forms a most interesting tale, unfolding, as ever, from a combination of episodic serendipity and persistent inquiry by a large group of hard-nosed scientific investigators.

Growth Hormone (GH)

There is nothing about the unusual syndrome of acromegaly to immediately suggest that growth hormone (GH) is out of control,

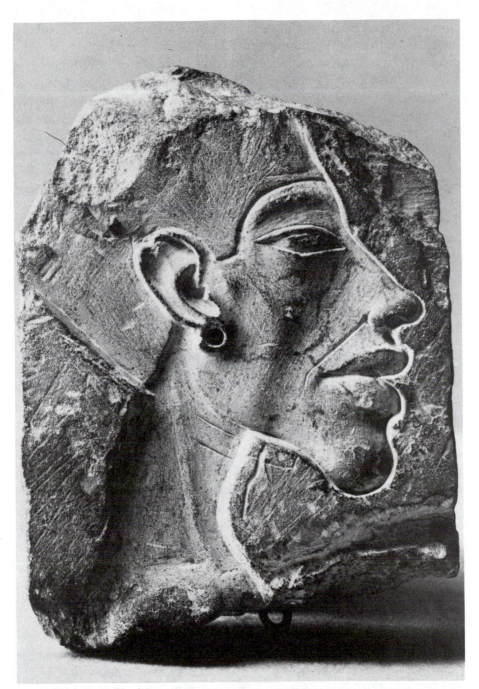

The Egyptian pharaoh Akhenaten who ruled from 1379–1362 B.C. may be the oldest known case of acromegaly.

leading to a perverse proliferation of soft tissues, bone, and cartilage. In this syndrome the excess growth hormone frequently originates from a pituitary tumor and then circulates to the liver. Growth hormone does not act directly on bones and soft tissues, but rather stimulates liver cells to produce growth factors (*somatomedins*) that do act directly on tissues. There are several types of somatomedins and they are the culprits in acromegaly—the reason why your shoes didn't fit anymore that fateful morning. Marie and others in the late nineteenth century knew that pituitary tumors were associated with acromegaly but they put the story together backward, proposing that the tumor destroyed normal pituitary tissue, thereby allowing a growth disorder to emerge. Marie and his colleagues were also unaware, although they discovered cases in paintings and sculpture as well as in the medical literature, that acromegaly was not a new disease but extended back into antiquity. (The oldest case may be Akhenaten, an ancient Egyptian pharaoh, who ruled from 1379-1362 B.C.)

The view that the anterior pituitary produced a growth factor got a big boost in 1909, when Cushing cured a 38-year-old South Dakota farmer of acromegaly by surgical removal of the pituitary tumor. This placed the idea that a growth hormone existed on much firmer ground. When, 12 years later, growth hormone was discovered in pituitary extracts, the existence of a growth-stimulating substance was widely accepted. Evans and Long carefully prepared an anterior pituitary extract from cows and injected it daily into rats. The results were astounding—the injected rats slowly began to get bigger than non-injected control rats. By the end of nine months, the rats given pituitary extract were gigantic in size, weighing several pounds. There was overgrowth of the skeleton and of most other tissues. Subsequently Evans produced an experimental model of acromegaly by giving pituitary extracts to dachshund dogs, producing a dramatic syndrome of soft tissue overgrowth.

It was a long way from this demonstration of growth-stimulating activity in pituitary extracts to the determination of the chemical structure of human growth hormone (HGH) 50 years later, in 1971. Many tedious chromatographic procedures and bioassays had to be undertaken in order to obtain chemically pure growth hormone from large quantities of animal or human pituitaries. Now we know that HGH is a peptide hormone composed of 191 amino acids that can be used to correct growth disorders in children. Because it can now be syn-

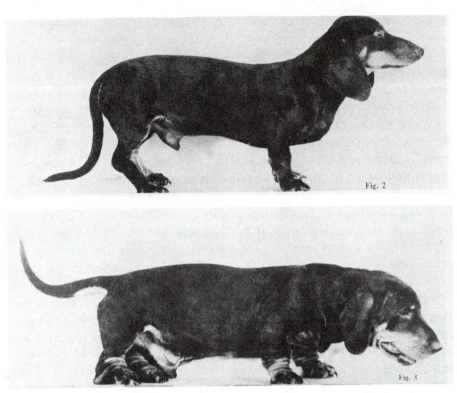

The effect of growth hormone on dachshund dogs is dramatically illustrated in these littermate brothers. The larger dog was given a daily injection of purified pituitary extract for a period of six months by Evans in 1931.

thesized in bacteria by using recombinant DNA techniques, the future supply of HGH should be plentiful.

The Gonadotropins (LH and FSH)

We now know that the anterior pituitary gland also secretes two hormones, called gonadotropins, which regulate the ovaries in females and the testes in males. Once again there is some economy here, because the hormones are identical in structure in both females and males, yet they play entirely different roles in the two settings. *Follicle-stimulating hormone* (FSH) induces maturation of follicles in the ovaries and of spermatozoa in the testes. *Luteinizing hormone* (LH) stimulates ovulation, estrogen secretion, and corpus luteum formation in the ovaries. Its role in the male is to stimulate testosterone production by the Leydig cells located in the interstitial tissue of the testes. The secretion of both LH and FSH from the pituitary is regulated from the hypothalamus by the same hormone, LH-releasing hormone (LHRH), which is controlled by nerve signals coming from the brain.

This detailed knowledge of the regulation of the gonads by the anterior pituitary has been acquired only during the past 60 years. Before that, important clues were available but none on which to found a definitive theory. By the beginning of the nineteenth century it was well known that certain female mammals, such as rabbits, ovulate and form corpora lutea only after coitus; but awareness that the act of coitus led to the release of gonadotropins from the pituitary obviously could not evolve until the gonadotropins were discovered in 1927.

As we have seen, the first awareness that the pituitary gland might be involved in the regulation of bodily functions began with the discovery of acromegaly by Marie. The observation that many female acromegalic patients stopped their menstrual cycles and that acromegalic men became impotent was a clue to the implication of the pituitary in the regulation of the ovaries and the testes—but went unrecognized. In 1900, a new syndrome was described by the French neurologist Babinski; upon the death of an obese 17-year-old girl with arrested sexual development autopsy revealed a large pituitary tumor and very small ovaries. A similar case of a 15-year-old boy with infantile testes and a pituitary tumor was published in 1901 by Fröhlich in Vienna. Neither of these patients had acromegaly; they represented a new disorder in which obesity and retarded sexual development were associated with a pituitary tumor.

Further experiments in animals provided unequivocal evidence that the pituitary gland produces hormones that control the gonads. Cushing and Aschner each showed that partial removal of the pituitary gland in dogs can lead to sexual infantilism and reduction in the size of the gonads. In 1922, Evans and Long noted that the same pituitary extracts that caused excessive growth in rats also caused enlargement of the ovaries as well as a disruption of the rat estrous cycles. Thus, gradually and inevitably, scientists stumbled onto the view that the pituitary might control the integrity of the ovaries and testes, possibly by an internal secretion. The laboratories of Smith and Zondek finally demonstrated in 1926 that daily implants of anterior pituitary glands from many different species would induce ovarian enlargement and precocious sexual maturation in rats and mice. The same implants also reversed the gonad atrophy resulting from removal of the pituitary gland. These exciting animal experiments left no doubt that the pituitary contains factors that act directly on the gonads.

Research in humans magnified these findings. Zondek discovered that the urine of pregnant women and of postmenopausal women both contained excessive quantities of hormones (gonadotropins) capable of stimulating the ovaries. (It was the gonadotropins isolated from the urine of postmenopausal women that recently led to the birth of septuplets in Southern California.) Noting that the urine of pregnant women produced primarily luteinizing activity and that the postmenopausal urine stimulated follicle development, he logically concluded that there existed two different gonadotropins.

Research over the next ten years demonstrated that there are in fact three gonadotropins. The urine of pregnant women contains human chorionic gonadotropin (HCG), which is made in the placenta and closely resembles LH in its action, whereas the urine of postmenopausal women contains follicle-stimulating hormone (FSH) and luteinizing hormone (LH) together. This results from the very high serum FSH and LH levels present in postmenopausal women, because the ovaries no longer secrete estrogen in amounts sufficient to keep the pituitary gonadotropins (LH and FSH) in check.

By the 1960s the gonadotropins LH, FSH, and HCG were all shown to be similar in structure, each composed of two peptide chains, called alpha and beta. The alpha peptide chains are identical for all three hormones and they each contain 89 amino acids. The differences among the gonadotropins are determined by the different amino acid sequences of their beta peptide chains. Thus each alpha-beta chain pair is biologically distinct.

The menstrual cycle is regulated in a complex fashion (see Figure 4-2). Estradiol produced by the ovaries during each cycle can suppress or stimluate LH and FSH release by the pituitary through feedback interaction. Estradiol and progesterone produced during the cycle are responsible for those changes in the uterine lining that lead to monthly bleeding. In the male, FSH regulates spermatogenesis and LH regulates the production of testosterone (which can feed back to suppress LH and FSH secretion by the pituitary).

Prolactin

It is rather surprising that a syndrome associating pituitary tumors with abnormal breast milk production (*galactorrhea*) in women was not discovered early on, as the syndrome is rather common today and most certainly existed at the time acromegaly was discovered. Nevertheless, there were no clues to suggest that the anterior pituitary made

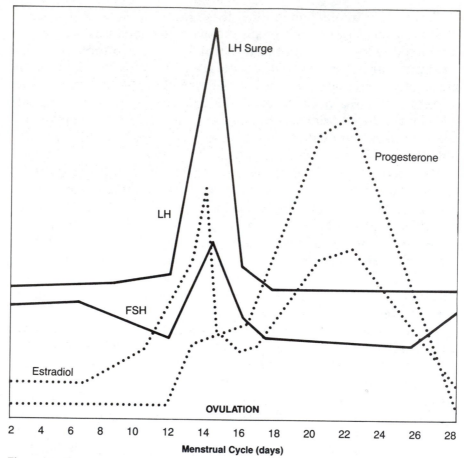

Figure 4-2. The gonadotropins LH and FSH regulate the menstrual cycle by stimulating estradiol secretion by the ovaries and by promoting mid-cycle ovulation. The LH surge releases the egg. Progesterone is produced by the corpus lutuem.

a breast-stimulating hormone until 1929, when several research groups noted by chance that injections of anterior pituitary extracts into rabbits or rats stimulated milk production in the mammary glands even when the ovaries were removed. This observation skewered the prevailing dogma of the time—that mammary gland development and milk production were controlled by the corpus luteum in the ovaries. The new pituitary hormone was called prolactin by Riddle. He noted that it not only stimulated breast milk production in mammals but was also responsible for crop milk production in pigeons and doves. That these birds feed their young a milk secretion from the crop gland had been discovered by Hunter in 1786, but no one had any idea that crop milk production was regulated by the pituitary gland until Riddle and his colleagues purified prolactin in the early 1930s. Prolactin, a pituitary hormone under the regulation of hypothalamic prolactin-releasing and prolactin-inhibiting factors can thus be seen as a universal hormone, conserved in the course of evolution for the provision of nutrition to the young.

It took decades to purify, isolate, and determine the chemical structure of prolactin—just as it had for the other anterior pituitary hormones—and required a multitude of new chromatography techniques and the development of more sensitive assays, such as the radioimmunoassay. The chemical structure of human prolactin as finally determined in the early 1970s turns out to be remarkably similar to human growth hormone. Prolactin is a peptide hormone containing one long sequence of 198 amino acids, whereas growth hormone contains 191 amino acids. Because of their similar structure, prolactin and growth hormone were very difficult to separate from each other chemically until sophisticated chromatography techniques could be developed. The considerable similarity between human prolactin and the prolactin molecules found in other vertebrates indicates the same conservation of useful chemical structures during evolution that we find for many other hormones.

In the human female, prolactin stimulates lactation following parturition, and in conjunction with other hormones it stimulates breast development during pregnancy. Although the synthesis of milk by breast cells is enhanced by prolactin, the actual ejection of milk from the milk sacs into the lobular ducts is controlled by the posterior pituitary hormone oxytocin, which stimulates the contraction of the milk sac lining to force milk into the ducts.

In the human male, prolactin seems to be a lost hormone, wandering around trying to find something to do—a pseudohormone without an apparent purpose. Prolactin in excess causes impotence in men and loss of menstrual function in women. In both men and women, life these days can go on without prolactin, since lactation is no longer necessary to feed small children. Perhaps prolactin was critical for survival in ancient times, and we are seeing only the vestigial tip of an evolutionary iceberg.

Thyroid-Stimulating Hormone (TSH)

It took a long time to discover that the thyroid gland was controlled by a hormone secreted by the pituitary gland. Around 1850 it was noticed in France that enlarged pituitary glands were associated with thyroid goiter in humans and animals; later the removal of the thyroid gland from rabbits was shown to produce pituitary enlargement. But this was an era of ignorance about glands and hormones, and consequently there was no intellectual framework into which such observations could be fitted. So what if the pituitary gland enlarged when the thyroid gland stopped producing thyroid hormone? How was anyone to know that the thyroid hormones T4 and T3 interact with the pituitary TSH-producing cells by a feedback loop, that when serum levels of T4 and T3 fall, the pituitary cells enlarge to produce more TSH (which in turn will do just what its name says—it will stimulate the thyroid gland to make more T4 and T3)? Seventy-five years went by until Smith finally showed (in 1926) that removal of the pituitary led to atrophy of the thyroid gland, which could then be restored with pituitary extracts.

The importance of the thyroid gland in regulating normal body functions became apparent during the nineteenth century after a series of interesting observations regarding certain pathological conditions. Cretinism in children had been noted for several centuries to be associated with enlargement of the thyroid gland (goiter). These children were retarded in growth and intelligence, soft and doughy to the touch, with enlarged protruding tongues and large goiters; short idiots with a very unusual appearance, they were usually seen in the Alps. In 1850 a description appeared of the first two cases of cretinism in which surgical exploration of the neck revealed that no thyroid gland was present. Thus cretinism seemed to occur in a setting where there was either no thyroid gland or a poorly functioning enlarged thyroid gland.

A new and unusual disorder was described in 1873 by Gull and designated by him as a cretinoid state occurring in adult women. His initial description of the first case vividly portrayed the overall picture: "Miss B, after the cessation of the catamenial period, became insensibly more and more languid, with general increase of bulk. The change went on from year to year, her face altering from oval to round, much like the full moon rising."

This was one of the first descriptions of the condition of *myxedema*, a chronic disorder primarily affecting older women. "Miss B became insensibly more languid" describes the condition exactly; it is an illness in which the patient slowly becomes cold, dry, and sluggish. The skin becomes puffy from the accumulation of proteins and fluids (hence the name myxedema by Ord in 1877), the voice hoarse, the hair lackluster, and the skin very dry. There is a slowing down, a lack of energy that comes over the patient. Gull and Ord reported ten cases of myxedema in the 1870s without awareness that the cause was a deficiency of thyroid hormone.

In the early 1880s the French surgeon Reverdin and the Swiss surgeon Kocher observed that, following the surgical removal of thyroid goiters, some patients languished and developed an illness remarkably similar to myxedema. It remained for Semon to hypothesize that cretinism, myxedema, and the postsurgical state were all disorders resulting from a loss of the thyroid gland and, finally, for Horsley to show that cretinism and myxedema could be produced in monkeys by removing the thyroid gland.

Murry discovered that myxedema could be cured by treating patients with extracts from sheep thyroid glands, a remarkable achievement and the first cure of an endocrine deficiency syndrome.

From all of this work it became clear that the integrity of the thyroid gland was essential for normal life. If the gland is deficient in early life, cretinism develops with severe mental retardation—which is why all newborn children are screened today for hypothyroidism. If the gland is deficient during adult life then myxedema develops.

The opposite syndrome also came to light during the nineteenth century in the writing of Parry, Graves, and Basedow, who described toxic goiter, a state where the thyroid gland enlarges and makes too much thyroid hormone. In contrast to myxedema, patients become hot and sweaty, with palpitations of the heart, nervousness, weight loss, and difficulty in sleeping. Too much thyroid hormone fires up the body into an overactive state just as too little leads to a hypoactive sluggish state. The serum level of thyroid hormone has to be just right, a fine balance between the extremes of myxedema and Graves' disease. This tight regulation of the serum thyroid hormone level is accomplished by TSH from the pituitary, and the cells that produce TSH are influenced by TRH from the hypothalamus and by the thyroid hormones T4 and T3 delivered to the blood by the thyroid gland.

A few clues began to filter in suggesting that the thyroid gland was not out there on its own, that TSH was in the wings imposing itself on the action. Rogowitsch observed that the removal of the thyroid gland from rabbits led to an enlargement of the pituitary gland. In 1912 Aschner noted that following the removal of the pituitary gland in dogs the thyroid gland became atrophic. But it was P. H. Smith who made the great breakthrough in a series of experiments beginning in

1926 by demonstrating that removal of rat pituitaries, which led to thyroid atrophy and a decreased metabolic rate, could be entirely corrected by pituitary implants or extracts.

From these initial observations that pituitary extracts contained thyroid-stimulating activity, it took nearly 50 more years of research to prove the existence of a separate TSH molecule, with its purification and chemical structure finally determined in the early 1970s. This was a tough hormone to purify because its structural similarity to LH and FSH made chemical separation very difficult until sophisticated chromatography techniques could be developed. TSH is a large peptide, like LH and FSH, with two subunit peptides designated alpha and beta, and some sugar side chains. The alpha-subunits of LH, FSH, and TSH are all identical; the molecules differ only in the beta-subunits and in the attached sugars. Thus, during evolution, nature has chosen to use some common alpha-subunits for 3 of the pituitary hormones in addition to very homologous structures for prolactin and growth hormone.

Adrenocortical-Stimulating Hormone (ACTH)

Attention was first focused on the adrenal glands in 1855, when Addison published his classic monograph entitled "On the Constitutional and Local Effects of Disease of the Supra-renal Capsules." He emphasized in his introduction that the rich blood and nerve supply of the adrenal glands (or supra-renal capsules, as they were known at the time), their early fetal development, their unimpaired integrity into old age, and their peculiar glandular structure "all point to the performance of some important office"; nevertheless, beyond the vague impression that the adrenal glands might be involved in the production of blood, Addison was "not aware that any modern authority has ventured to assign them any special function or influence whatsoever."

The "important office" performed by the adrenal glands turned out to be the preservation of life itself, for Addison showed that destruction of the adrenal glands leads to an illness causing patients to wither away and die. Initially there is a gradual falling off of general health, with a peculiar discoloration of the skin, which "may be said to present a dingy or smoky appearance, or various tints or shades of deep amber or chestnut brown." Weakness and fatigue are accompanied by loss of appetite and occasional vomiting or stomach pains. There is a wasting away, with weight loss and a fall in blood pressure; "the pulse becomes smaller and weaker, and without any special complaint of pain or uneasiness, the patient at length gradually sinks and expires."

This once uniformly fatal illness results from any disease process that destroys the adrenal glands and thereby deprives patients of cortisol to support their general well-being (including the appetite) and aldosterone to support blood pressure (by retaining salt in the body). Of course Addison didn't know about cortisol and aldosterone at the time of his discovery, for there was no theory of internal secretion of hormones at that time and no framework for thinking about chemical messengers. Initially, Addison felt that the adrenal glands had a special function of their own in body economy, but eventually he modified his view to the notion that diseased adrenal glands may affect the neighboring autonomic nerve centers and thereby have an indirect effect on the body via the nervous system—which was the standard way of thinking about the glands during the nineteenth century. Then, as now, thinking was warped by tradition, and so it was another 40 years before the idea of chemical messengers would be introduced, even though clues to their existence were staring everyone in the face much earlier.

After the initial monograph on what came to be known as "Addison's disease" appeared in 1855, other investigators found that complete removal of the adrenal glands in animals invariably led to death of the animal, thus proving that the adrenals were essential for life in many different species. Still there were no hints that the pituitary was involved in regulation of the adrenals. That awareness came slowly.

Turn-of-the-century experiments on dogs led to the realization that removal of the pituitary gland could lead to atrophy of the adrenal gland cortex. Simmonds noticed that patients whose pituitary gland was destroyed by disease developed adrenal atrophy. During the 1920s Smith and his co-workers opened up a whole new vision of adrenal regulation by performing a set of experiments on tadpoles and rats. They first removed the pituitary from these animals and then demonstrated that the atrophy of the adrenal gland could be reversed by injection of extracts from the pituitary glands of cows. These experiments proved that pituitary extracts contain a substance capable of stimulating the adrenal gland, but debate ensued about the nature of the stimulating substance. Some argued for the existence of a separate ACTH molecule and others argued that growth hormone or prolactin stimulated the adrenal gland.

Collip and others cleared up this impasse during the 1930s by careful purification procedures on pituitary extracts and thereby established the independent identity of ACTH. There still remained the tasks of improving the assay for ACTH and achieving some further advances in purification in order finally to have its chemical structure determined. That it is secreted in pulses from the pituitary mostly during the early morning hours is known. Many of the other pituitary hormones are also secreted episodically, but the physiologic reason for this secretion pattern is not known.

New Vistas

The six anterior pituitary hormones we have discussed are shown in Table 4-1. All of these hormones are made inside cells in the pituitary gland from precursor molecules. These cells are specialized to produce just the right hormones, whose synthesis and release into the circulation are regulated from the brain by the hypothalamic-releasing hormones. These specialized cells are also regulated by feedback signals from the target glands so that cortisol, for example, will suppress ACTH production in the ACTH-producing cells. The precursor molecules, or prohormones, are clipped by enzymes to the final hormones before release from the pituitary cells.

The most interesting prohormone in the pituitary gland is a very large molecule and contains, in addition to the amino acid sequence for ACTH, the amino acid sequences for two other peptides called beta-lipotropin (beta-LPH) and beta-endorphin. Thus ACTH, beta-LPH, and beta-endorphin are all produced in the same cell from the same precursor prohormone and are released into the circulation during times of acute stress. ACTH stimulates cortisol and aldosterone release from the adrenal gland, while beta-endorphin is one of the internal narcotics (opioid peptides) that presumably modulate pain thresholds in the body and brain. The role of beta-LPH is not yet known. It is possible that some of the pituitary hormones like beta-endorphin circulate back to the brain to influence sensory perceptions or other brain functions. The discovery in the anterior pituitary of a precursor to ACTH and an opioid peptide has opened new vistas of thinking about the interaction between the pituitary gland and the brain. We will discuss these in more detail in the last chapter.

5

THE MYSTERIOUS
PINE CONE

■

That which is interesting does not always coincide with that which is important.
—Ancient proverb

Imagine yourself—if you haven't already done so—as the Supreme Being, the creator of the universe some 20 billion years ago. You start things out with a huge explosion, something to rattle the cosmos right down to its marrow. As the debris from this big bang goes swirling off into an infinite vortex of empty space you decide to precipitate out a few galaxies complete with stars, planets, moons, comets, and all sorts of unusual phenomena to keep everyone guessing about your ultimate intentions. You allow for the evolution of a strange species called humans located on an even stranger planet called Earth. Just for laughs, perhaps as an entertaining diversion from your basic plan, you decide to endow your creation with a mysterious gland, located in the center of the brain, thereby giving generation after generation of curious scientists a challenging focus of intellectual activity. You give them something interesting to chew on without, of course, revealing the importance of the structure in your overall design. What you have inadvertently created here is a scientist's nightmare, an inscrutable organ that has come to be known as the pineal gland.

The pineal gland sits in the center of the brain, overlooking the aqueduct of Sylvius, and its function has baffled physicians and philosophers alike throughout the centuries. It is small, about the size of a pea, and is shaped like the pine cone from which it derives its name.

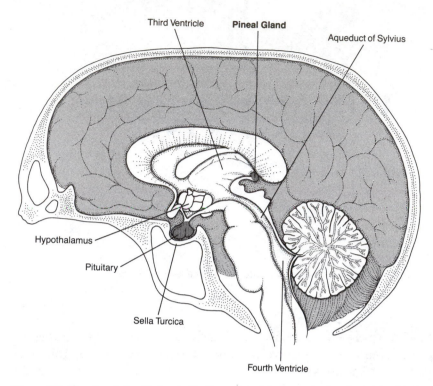

Third Ventricle   **Pineal Gland**   Aqueduct of Sylvius

Hypothalamus

Pituitary

Sella Turcica

Fourth Ventricle

Figure 5-1. The pineal gland is located in the center of the brain on the edge of the third ventricle.

The pineal gland today is regarded much as the pituitary gland was in the nineteenth century—a gland without an apparent purpose, a gland lost on its way into an evolutionary black hole, perhaps a vestige of a part of the body useful in times past. It remains the last endocrine gland in the human body whose function is not known; scientific investigators are now, however, closing in on the answer.

Galen, about 1,800 years ago—and the Greek anatomists before him—knew about the existence of the pineal gland (see Figure 5-1). The pineal sits perched right in the center of things at the gateway between the third and fourth ventricles of the brain. Cerebrospinal fluid flows from the two lateral ventricles into the third ventricle and then on to the fourth ventricle through the aqueduct of Sylvius, like water moving through the Carquinez Strait from the Sacramento Delta to the San Francisco Bay. The Greek anatomist Herophilus concluded that the pineal gland was not just sitting there on the shore of the third ventricle gazing out into the brain, listening to waves of cerebrospinal fluid crashing in on the ventricle walls, but rather that it was a sphincter whose job was to regulate the flow of thought out of the lateral ventricles. By the seventeenth century, the view was that the pineal regulated the flow of cerebrospinal fluid through the ventricles and in particular through the Sylvian aqueduct, but this theory had gradually been abandoned by the end of the nineteenth century. Several cases of early puberty in very young boys who were found to have tumors in the pineal gland led to a new theory that the pineal in some way regulates the testes and ovaries.

The French philosopher René Descartes published the first textbook of human physiology in the mid-seventeenth century. His theory of the pineal gland is illustrated in Figure 5-2. In this formulation the body is like a machine, with its mechanics controlled by a "rational soul" situated in the pineal gland. Objects in the real world are visualized through the eyes, and this information is transferred through the brain by connections to the pineal gland, where the information is processed by the rational soul. The pineal also accumulated "animal spirits" from the arterial circulation and then released these spirits into the ventricles; from there they traveled through hollow nerves to the muscles. Descartes' scheme of the pineal gland as a neuroendocrine transducer that converts signals from the eyes into humors in the body is surprisingly close to our view of the pineal today—namely that the pineal receives nerve signals originating in the retina of the eye and secretes a unique hormone in response to these signals.

Very little experimental information about the pineal gland began to accumulate until early in the twentieth century, when Holmgren in Sweden discovered that the pineal gland of frogs and other cold-blooded vertebrates looks just like cone cells of the retina under the light microscope; this suggested that in these animals the pineal may function as a third eye by acting as a photoreceptor for light. The pineal of the frog, located just under the skin on the back of the head, has recently been shown to convert certain wavelengths of light into nerve impulses, thus verifying Holmgren's hypothesis that in lower vertebrates the pineal acts like a third eye. It is not a bad idea to have a photosensitive pineal body on the back of your head when someone is trying to sneak up on you from the rear. Unfortunately, in mammals like us, the pineal is located deep in the center of the brain and therefore cannot transduce light directly.

The pineal came to be generally viewed as an evolutionary leftover in mammals until Lerner's landmark discovery in 1958 of the pineal hormone, *melatonin*. The clue to this discovery had actually been buried

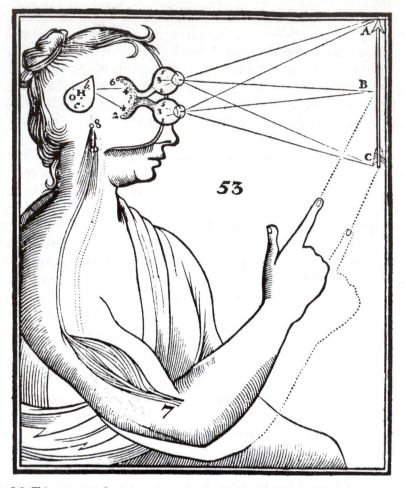

Figure 5-2. This seventeenth century engraving depicts the regulation of the body by the pineal gland according to Descartes' theory that the pineal is the seat of the rational soul, receiving signals from the eyes and sending signals to the muscles through hollow tubes.

deep in the literature for 40 years, ever since experiments by McCord and Allen showed that extracts prepared from the pineal glands of cattle would lighten the color of tadpoles' skin when added to the fluid in which tadpoles were swimming. The tadpoles were probably just out for a nice afternoon swim when scientists threw some pineal extracts into their pool; then they noticed their skin color starting to disappear—a midafternoon blanch beyond one's control. As disconcerting as these experiments may have been for the integrity of the tadpoles, they strongly suggested that mammalian pineal extracts contained a substance that could directly affect the melanin-containing cells of frog skin.

The Melatonin Hypothesis

Lerner and his co-workers at Yale took a continued interest in the skin-lightening effects of pineal extracts. In an effort to isolate the substance in the pineal gland responsible for blanching tadpoles, they first developed a sensitive photometric assay from frog skin and then plunged into processing massive quantities of pineal glands obtained from cattle in a fashion reminiscent of Schally and Guillemin and their hypothalamic extracts from millions of pigs and sheep. Over a four-year period Lerner processed the pineal glands of over 200,000 cattle and in 1958 finally isolated the factor that lightens melanocytes in the skin of frogs. They called the new factor melatonin because it stimulated the clustering of melanin pigment granules within the melanocyte cells. (They showed that the structure of melatonin was a unique biological molecule containing a ring with an attached methyl group CH_3 as shown in Figure 5-3). Research by Axelrod and others added new information—melatonin can be synthesized from the amino acid tryptophan through a series of steps catalyzed by enzymes present only in the pineal gland.

At last the pineal gland was on the map as an organ capable of making the unique compound melatonin in mammals and other vertebrates. Finding a new substance in mammal pineal glands that blanched the skin of tadpoles and frogs was important, but the key

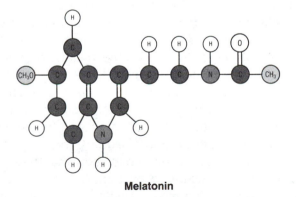

Melatonin

Figure 5-3. Melatonin, a unique molecule discovered by Lerner at Yale, contains an indole ring with an attached methyl (CH_3-) group. It is synthesized from the amino acid tryptophan.

question remained: What was the melatonin doing in mammals? Melatonin did not blanch the skin of mammals, so obviously its action lay elsewhere.

Nineteen sixty-one was a big year for melatonin. First, observations by Kappers in the Netherlands clarified the anatomy of the pineal gland in mammals. He found that the pineal gland of the rat loses all of its direct connections with the brain soon after birth. Consequently, there is no direct nerve pathway between the pineal and the central nervous system (in amphibians and fish, the pineal is connected by the pineal nerve to the brain). Thus, in rats and other mammals, information cannot be delivered to the pineal gland directly from the central nervous system. More importantly, Kappers showed that the pineal gland in rats is loaded with nerves of the sympathetic nervous system originating in the superior cervical ganglion in the neck. The existence of a nerve pathway connecting the retina of the eye to the superior ganglion was the next discovery. Light signals received by the retina could influence the pineal gland through this path (see Figure 5-4).

Still others discovered (by electron microscopy) that the sympathetic nerves to the pineal gland terminate directly on the pineal cells that produce melatonin. Like a hormone, melatonin is released into the circulation and possibly into the cerebrospinal fluid, where it could conceivably influence brain function. The regulation of pineal cells by the sympathetic nervous system is remarkably similar to the process by which the release of epinephrine from adrenal medulla cells is controlled. The pineal gland, like the adrenal medulla, can be viewed as a neuroendocrine transducer; that is, nerve signals from the sympathetic nervous system are converted into a hormone signal by the pineal cells.

The discovery of the pineal hormone melatonin and of a nerve pathway from the eyes to the pineal gland was not yet the whole story, as continued research revealed. In 1961, Fiske at Wellesley College discovered that when female rats are exposed to several weeks of continuous light their pineal glands decrease in weight and their ovaries simultaneously get larger. Wurtman and his colleagues confirmed these observations and went on to show that the same enlarging effect on rat ovaries was achieved by removing the pineal gland. He further demonstrated that pineal extracts and melatonin could both decrease the weight of rat ovaries and simultaneously slow the estrous cycle. These experiments were followed by studies which showed that

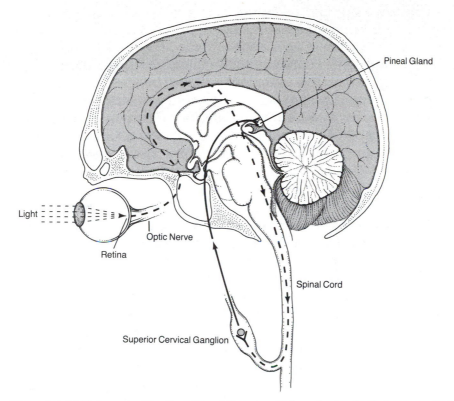

Light

Optic Nerve

Retina

Pineal Gland

Spinal Cord

Superior Cervical Ganglion

Figure 5-4. Light is received by the retina of the eye, which sends signals along a sympathetic nerve pathway to the superior cervical ganglion; from here the signals are transmitted to the pineal gland.

when rats are exposed to continuous light, the pineal enzyme responsible for synthesizing melatonin markedly decreases in activity—and markedly increases when the animals are left in continuous darkness. Over a 24-hour period in which the environmental light was alternated to simulate a natural day-night cycle, the enzyme activity was low during the 12-hour light period and maximum during the 12-hour dark period. It all adds up to the "melatonin hypothesis" of Wurtman and Axelrod—that melatonin is a hormone whose synthesis and release by the pineal gland is controlled by light signals arriving at the retina in a day-night cyclic biological rhythm, and that melatonin regulates gonadal function and possibly other physiologic effects in mammals.

Very sensitive assays for melatonin became available in the 1970s and made possible detailed studies of the daily rhythms exhibited by the hormone in various body fluids, as well as an assessment of the first part of the melatonin hypothesis. All vertebrates studied so far show a daily rhythm in melatonin secretion, marked by much higher blood or urine levels of melatonin at night (or during a dark period) than during the day. This biological rhythm appears to be universal in all animals with pineal glands. Exposing the animal to continuous light or removing the pineal gland breaks the pattern, leaving a low background level of melatonin in the circulation (which comes from cells in the retina and intestine). Green light appears to be much more effective in abolishing the melatonin daily rhythm than are other wavelengths.

The suppression of pineal melatonin secretion by continuous light can be overcome by stress severe enough to release epinephrine from the adrenal medulla. The epinephrine in turn stimulates melatonin release from the pineal, leading to the conjecture that melatonin may be a stress hormone that in some way plays a role in adaptation to stressful conditions. Some melatonin may be secreted directly into the cerebrospinal fluid, although the evidence to date suggests that most of the melatonin is secreted from the pineal cells directly into the bloodstream. Once secreted into the bloodstream, melatonin is metabolized very rapidly in the liver into a form allowing excretion into the urine. Melatonin also appears to be able to pass from the circulation into the brain and the cerebrospinal fluid without difficulty, suggesting that it may play a role in the regulation of brain function.

We humans, like other mammals, secrete most of our melatonin at night between 11:00 P.M. and 7:00 A.M. and then switch it back off during the day. This whole sequence of events—from the retina, to the superior cervical ganglion, to the pineal gland—is controlled by the sympathetic nervous system. Light suppresses and darkness enhances nerve signals from the superior cervical ganglion to the pineal gland, where melatonin synthesis and release are promoted. This daily biological rhythm is controlled by changes in the amount of external light and is abolished if the nerve tracts are cut, the pineal is removed, or animals are exposed to an unchanging amount of light. When mammals are exposed to continuous darkness, however, a fascinating event occurs: Melatonin secretion continues to oscillate in a daily rhythm, indicating that in addition to an external light-dark regulation cycle there exists an internal daily melatonin rhythm controlled by a biological clock somewhere in the brain and linked to the pineal gland.

As more and more detailed quantitative studies of the pineal gland are performed, the gland appears increasingly complex.

What Does the Pineal Gland Do?

Thus far we have ascertained that the pineal gland secretes melatonin in a light-regulated daily cycle, which is controlled through the sympathetic nervous system in mammals and by direct photostimulation in lower organisms. The pineal gland in amphibians and fish is a photoreceptor located near the skin surface and transforms light directly into a nerve signal that is transmitted directly to the brain by the pineal nerve. It acts as a third eye, a photoreceptor that sends signals to the brain from an environmental light stimulus. In birds the pineal is a photoendocrine transducer; it receives direct light signals but then converts this information into a hormonal signal like melatonin.

In mammals light is received by the eye, which transmits a nerve signal to the superior cervical ganglion and from there to the pineal gland to regulate melatonin output; it is a neuroendocrine transducer, receiving a nerve signal from the superior cervical ganglion and converting it into a hormone signal. The pineal has undergone an evolutionary change from a photoreceptor to a photoendocrine transducer to a neuroendocrine transducer, but has maintained a responsiveness to environmental light stimuli. At a certain stage of evolution, melatonin was introduced to act as a hormone secreted by the pineal into the circulation.

At this point it is important to ask: What in the world does the melatonin *do*, and does melatonin (as suggested in the melatonin hypothesis) really mediate any or all of the physiologic effects of the pineal gland? Does the pineal gland really do anything in humans, or is it just lying around wondering why everyone is getting so excited; why research careers in pineal physiology are being mapped out and symposia on pineal function are being planned; why pinealogists are starting to appear on earth; when it may decide to spring loose the grant-shattering truth one day in the form of an official statement: "The melatonin's just a cruel joke, a vestige from bygone years. I'm just lying around now doing nothing, enjoying all the attention." On the other hand, the joke could eventually be on the pineal skeptics, that legion of internists, physiologists, and endocrinologists who cringe at the word "pineal," who show that trace of contempt when you ask them at the cocktail party what the pineal gland does—the same legion who would have been sneering at the pituitary gland 100 years ago. The pineal gland and melatonin may yet turn out to be important, perhaps in the regulation of fundamental biological rhythms centered in the brain. To consider the role of the pineal we will first evaluate studies of lower animals and then compare these results with the data from human studies.

Pineal Function in Animals

The Syrian hamster is not the kind of animal that generally inspires confidence in your research program, as rats, mice, guinea pigs, or monkeys do. And yet it is the Syrian hamster that has allowed critical breakthroughs in understanding pineal physiology, because it is an animal whose reproductive pattern is seasonal, so that its fertility can occur only at certain times of the year. The Syrian hamster is infertile during the winter months and becomes sexually activated in early spring, which, together with the short gestation period, insures that the birth of offspring will take place in the late spring. Mammals and other species living in temperate regions of the earth, where there are marked annual changes in temperature and in the availability of food, have evolved elaborate mechanisms to insure that the offspring will be born in the spring. The reproductive cycle of the Syrian hamster is regulated by the pineal gland through the seasonal changes in the day-night photoperiod.

When Syrian hamsters are studied under conditions of natural photoperiods through the year, their reproductive cycle is observed to go through the phases shown in Figure 5-5. When exposure to light drops below a certain level per day in late September, the reproductive system in both male and female hamsters collapses. Testes shrink in size and weight and their output of testosterone falls; ovarian function similarly declines. The hamsters gradually slide into a sexually dormant phase, unaware that the decreased light period has fired up their pineal gland output of melatonin, which in turn has decreased their pituitary output of luteinizing hormone (LH) and follicle-stimulating hormone (FSH). They probably aren't too happy about this gradual deterioration of the sexual scene; their mates don't seem quite so attractive anymore, so what else is there to do but hibernate, lie low until the reproductive system spontaneously regenerates in early spring.

There is good evidence that the pineal gland mediates the gonadal regression induced by the short light cycle in Syrian hamsters, prob-

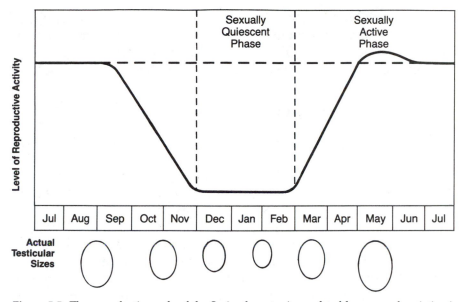

Figure 5-5. The reproductive cycle of the Syrian hamster is regulated by seasonal variation in the amount of daylight through the pineal gland.

ably by secretion of melatonin. If the pineal gland is removed or if its sympathetic nerve supply is interrupted, then testicular atrophy does *not* occur when the light cycle is shortened; a functioning pineal gland is necessary in order for hamsters to shift into a quiescent phase of reproduction. The gonadal atrophy induced in Syrian hamsters by a short light cycle can be simulated by giving daily melatonin injections in the late afternoon; the pineal gland thus appears to regulate the reproductive system of hamsters by means of the hormone melatonin, which is released from the pineal in the absence of light. Melatonin must be given in a late afternoon daily dose to induce gonad suppression; if it is given at other times or continuously delivered, no gonad regression occurs.

It's a somewhat different story in rats. When the pineal gland is removed from rats, the daily rhythms of melatonin levels in the plasma and urine are abolished, and the total daily melatonin excretion is reduced by over 80 percent—but the dramatic effects on reproduction seen in the hamster do not appear. The pineal gland in the rat may not be as critical to reproduction as it is in the hamster. It may perform different functions in different animals; however, in all of the mammals studied thus far, including humans, melatonin excretion from the pineal shows a daily rhythm marked by increased excretion at night. The enzyme activity responsible for the synthesis of melatonin from tryptophan in pineal cells also shows the same daily rhythm, a rhythm that can be abolished by removing the sympathetic nerve supply to the pineal gland.

Pineal Function in Humans

We come down then to the question: What is the role of the pineal gland in humans? This remains a mystery even today; it is not possible to say with any degree of certainty just exactly what the pineal is doing in humans other than secreting melatonin at night on a cyclic basis. The data that are available, however, are worth examining and may serve as a basis for speculation.

Throughout the eons the pineal gland, sitting as it does in the center of the brain, has been the subject of some rather resourceful speculation. The ancient Greeks viewed the pineal as a device to regulate the flow of thought out of the brain ventricles—an idea that Galen replaced with the notion that the pineal was like a lymph gland. This is a remarkably modern notion, considering that Galen was sitting there without a microscope to show him that the pineal indeed contained glandlike structures. In the seventeenth century Descartes, as we noted, conceived of the pineal as the seat of the rational soul, receiving input from the eyes and then regulating the body by allowing animal humors to flow to the muscles. (He would have been pleased to know that melatonin secretion by the pineal gland can be regulated by input from the eyes.) These ideas were followed by several hundred more years of wild speculation about the function of the pineal gland— with no experimental data in sight, as the blind led the deaf through a myriad of unsupported theories.

Then in 1898 the German physician Otto Huebner published the case of a very young boy who experienced early puberty (an event called "precocious puberty") and who was found to have a tumor of the pineal gland. Since then many cases of precocious puberty, occurring almost exclusively in young boys, have been reported in association with pineal tumors.

Because puberty is normally initiated by the activation of LH and FSH in the pituitary by the hypothalamic-releasing hormone LHRH, the view has developed that somehow pineal gland tumors lead to activation of the pituitary hormones. Recent studies have shown that some of these tumors make a hormone that is very similar to LH; in these cases the LH-like hormone stimulates Leydig cells in the testes to make testosterone, which in turn causes precocious puberty to occur. There is no evidence to date either that the tumors produce an excess of melatonin or that they destroy the pineal gland and thus lead to a paucity of melatonin. No direct link between the pineal gland and the pituitary gland via melatonin or other pineal hormones has yet been discovered in humans. Some of these pineal tumors could conceivably cause a compression of the hypothalamus, leading to release of LHRH and thus causing precocious puberty, but this remains to be established.

After Lerner discovered the existence of melatonin and Kappers showed the pineal gland in mammals to be directly connected to the brain only through the sympathetic nervous system originating in the superior cervical ganglion, Wurtman and Axelrod developed a hypothesis to explain a number of phenomena observed in lower mammals such as rats and hamsters. Their hypothesis proposes that melatonin is a hormone secreted from the pineal gland and regulated by the sympathetic nervous system, which acts at distant sites to regulate reproduction. Does the melatonin hypothesis or something similar to it apply to human beings? During the 1970s some very specific and sensitive assays for melatonin and its metabolic derivatives were developed, allowing detailed evaluation of melatonin secretion in humans.

Humans do show daily variation in serum melatonin levels similar to that shown in other mammals—low levels during the day and high levels at night. Several lines of evidence indicate that the rate of melatonin secretion from the pineal gland in humans is controlled by the sympathetic nervous system. First, the sympathetic nerve blocker propranolol markedly reduces nocturnal melatonin levels, indicating that the stimulus to the pineal gland to release melatonin is transmitted by sympathetic nerves. Second, patients who have neck fractures lose their capacity to secrete melatonin, because the nerve supply from the superior cervical ganglion to the pineal gland is disrupted. Finally, patients with rare diseases of the sympathetic nerves also lose their normal daily variation in melatonin secretion.

What is the relationship between light received by the eyes and the secretion of melatonin by the pineal gland? Early studies in humans failed to demonstrate that light received by the retina would suppress nocturnal melatonin secretion as it does in rats and hamsters. More recent studies using bright artificial light have demonstrated convincingly that nocturnal melatonin secretion can be suppressed by light of sufficient intensity. Humans need more intense light to suppress melatonin secretion than do other mammals. Studies in blind humans give variable melatonin secretion patterns; in a recent study of ten blind persons, six subjects showed an abnormal pattern of melatonin secretion, with peak melatonin production occurring at times other than at night, and four subjects showed a normal melatonin profile.

Serum melatonin levels in the blood are obviously influenced by the light-dark cycle to form a fundamental biological rhythm linked to seasonal variations in the day and night cycle, but, even without light input from the eye, the pineal secretion of melatonin will have its own internal biological rhythm, probably regulated from the brain via the sympathetic nerve tract. The pineal appears to be linked to other natural and biological rhythms; for example, serum melatonin levels are influenced by the sleep-wake cycle and the menstrual cycle. Recent studies have shown that with age there is a steady decline of morning serum levels of melatonin, and the prominent nocturnal rise in serum melatonin seen in young persons is also markedly diminished in old age. Melatonin secretion by the pineal gland is thus flattened over time, abolishing the daily rhythm and leaving behind a rather monotonous melatonin profile.

The important question is: What does melatonin do in *humans*? If we could answer that, we would be able to determine what the pineal gland does. Whatever it does is probably mediated by melatonin or one of the more obscure peptides (such as vasotocin) or indoles (such as methoxytryptophol) that are occasionally released from the pineal gland in addition to melatonin. Of course, the pineal gland could be secreting a critically important compound, not yet identified, that failed to show up in Lerner's pineal extracts from 200,000 cattle. At present, however, most investigators feel that the primary function of the pineal gland is to secrete melatonin in response to signals coming in from the eye and brain along the sympathetic nerve fibers from the superior cervical ganglion. In this view, the role of the pineal gland in human physiology, if any, is determined by the role of melatonin. Consequently, everyone has been searching for the role and site of action of melatonin.

Because pineal tumors have been associated with early puberty in humans, and because melatonin appears to regulate reproduction in some mammalian species such as hamsters, the emphasis of melatonin research has been to investigate its effects on human reproduction

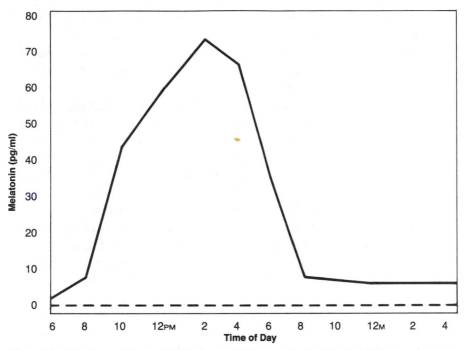

Figure 5-6. Plasma melatonin levels before (solid line) and after (dashed line) removal of the pineal gland in a 17-year-old boy with a pineal tumor.

and puberty. One intriguing observation is that in northern Finland most conceptions appear to take place during the summer, at the time of the long light cycle, so that the children are born the following spring. Of course, this need not have anything to do with suppression of melatonin by light and the consequent increase in fertility. A serious downturn in mating may occur during the winter, a frosting over of the primal sex drives until the following Midsummer Eve, or possibly just a problem of poor logistics, with everyone groping around in the dark—although the sharp upturn of births nine months after the New York City blackout in the mid-70s would tend to refute this conjecture!

An interesting experiment was reported in 1979 from the United Kingdom in which serum melatonin levels were measured in 51 healthy schoolchildren, ages 11 to 14 years. This study found a marked fall in the melatonin level in boys as they moved from prepuberty into puberty, just before the pubertal rise in LH, FSH, and testosterone. The investigators concluded that melatonin could play an important role in the regulation of the onset of human puberty. Unfortunately, this fall in melatonin secretion at the time of puberty was not seen in two other studies published in 1982, in which 24-hour serum melatonin profiles and daily urine excretion of the melatonin metabolite, 6-hydroxymelatonin, were carefully measured in prepubertal, pubertal, and adult subjects. So the role of melatonin in the onset of human puberty is still up in the air.

In 1983 the *New England Journal of Medicine* reported an unusual case of a 17-year-old boy with a pineal tumor. Before surgical removal of the pineal gland and tumor, a 24-hour melatonin profile was determined from plasma samples drawn every two hours, as shown in Figure 5-6. The profile showed the normal nocturnal rise in plasma melatonin. After surgery, melatonin levels were undetectable, demonstrating that in humans all of the melatonin measured in the blood comes from the pineal gland. Unfortunately, no studies of the patient's reproductive system were done, so we don't know if the absence of his pineal gland has had any discernible physiological impact, although the investigators did report that the boy is doing well 16 months after surgery.

What do we know then about the function of the mysterious pineal gland in humans? We know for sure that the pineal gland is a neuro-transducer that receives nerve signals from the sympathetic system and secretes melatonin into the bloodstream in a cyclic biological rhythm. It acts like a biological clock, but we don't know what kind of time it is keeping or what the melatonin is doing. Many hormones in the hypothalamus, the pituitary, and probably elsewhere in the brain demonstrate daily oscillations that are important to their functioning. Perhaps in time we will learn how the pineal rhythm is linked to other rhythms in the brain and thereby gain a more complete understanding of its role in human physiology. At this point only the most ardent skeptic (the one who chokes on his martini olive when the word "pineal" is mentioned) would believe that the pineal gland will turn out to have no role in humans, and be revealed in the end as merely a vestige of the third eye.

6

IT'S A GIRL

■

But on the very big matters, the times requiring exactly the right hunch, the occasions when the survival of human beings is in question, I would trust that X chromosome and worry about the Y.
                                        —Lewis Thomas, *The Youngest Science*

Whether or not you agree with the suggestion by Lewis Thomas that the male Y chromosome has led to plenty of trouble in the world, he does raise interesting questions about the role of sex chromosomes in male and female behavior. Do the X and Y chromosomes contain regions of DNA that code for female and male personality traits? Do there exist female brains and male brains? How do the X and Y chromosomes lead to female and male sexual development? We will attempt to confront these and other important questions about sexual differentiation in this chapter.

Just about ten years ago Julianne Imperato-McGinley and her colleagues first described an unusual syndrome observed in the rural village of Salinas in the southwestern region of the Dominican Republic: Children raised as girls turned into boys at puberty. The affected individuals are referred to by the villagers as *guevedoce* ("penis at 12 years of age") or alternatively as *machihembra* ("first woman, then man"). Here is a disconcerting Kafka-like metamorphosis if ever there was one: You're cruising along on the distaff side of life in a rural Caribbean village, being reared as a girl, thinking that it's nice to be a girl in a world where men are constantly botching things up, when slowly the horrifying awareness that you're becoming one of them, that someone has got your assignment all wrong, begins to unfold.

Gradually, as your breasts fail to develop and your body unravels along strikingly masculine lines, you no longer feel like a woman; in fact you feel like a man. You begin to dress like a man and take a sexual interest in women, eventually settling down to live happily as a married male. This is the fate of the vast majority of persons with the guevedoce syndrome.

This syndrome is extremely important not only to those who live through it, but also to researchers who are interested in sexual development. It results from a defect in the metabolism of the male hormone testosterone, and knowledge of this defect has led to a more complete understanding of sexual differentiation, the process by which girls become girls and boys become boys. To move beyond the Adam and Eve creation myth it is necessary to examine in detail what is known about the extraordinary process of sexual assignment whereby the genetically directed blueprint for gender plays itself out along a highly regulated developmental and metabolic line. Mistakes in this process unfortunately lead to aberrations like the guevedoce syndrome, but through these mistakes of nature much has been learned about the mechanisms that regulate sexual differentiation.

The program for sex designation begins at fertilization, when a spermatozoon unites with an egg, each supplying 23 separate strands of DNA, called chromosomes, to form a fertilized egg with 46 chromosomes. Two are sex chromosomes and, when things are going well, these two strands of DNA determine whether you turn out to be a boy or a girl. There are two different types of sex chromosomes—X and Y. The spermatozoa can contain either an X or a Y chromosome but unfertilized eggs contain only an X chromosome; the fertilized egg will therefore contain either two X chromosomes (XX), leading to female sexual development, or an X and Y chromosome (XY), resulting in male development. The pairing of these two sex chromosomes contains all of the genetic information necessary to set in motion your precise embryonic development into a girl or a boy.

Gonadal sex is determined by genetic sex; that is, the genetic pairing XX codes for the creation of ovaries in the developing embryo, whereas XY codes for the development of testes. Occasionally things go wrong in this transformation and a true hermaphrodite is produced—a person who has both ovarian and testicular tissue present at the same time, an ambiguity that is fortunately not common.

Even if your genetic sex assignment and your gonadal sex development have moved along a flawless pathway you are still not home free

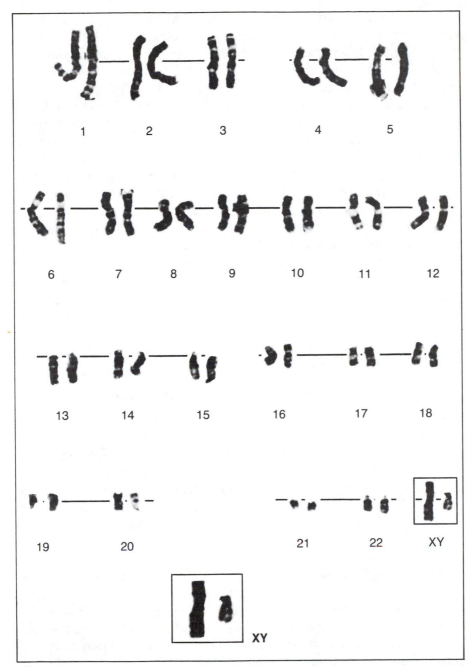

There are 46 chromosomes in human cells, which include 22 paired chromosomes plus the X and Y sex chromosomes. Female cells carry two X chromosomes and male cells carry an X and a Y chromosome.

with an unambiguous final assignment. Murphy's Law—"If anything can go wrong it will"—can still come into play during fetal development. The sex assignment of a child depends upon the appearance of the external genitalia at birth; this is called the *sex phenotype* and usually corresponds to the genetic sex and the gonadal sex. When ovaries are present, the fetus will usually turn out to be female. For males things are not quite so straightforward. The testes secrete two hormones, testosterone and müllerian regression hormone, both necessary to transform the embryo into a male. If these hormones are absent or don't work properly, the fetus will develop as a female; when testosterone doesn't work at all (because its receptors are absent) the child will appear at birth to be a normal female, even though it has a male genetic sex of XY and two testes concealed in the abdomen. A genetic male child that has external genitalia with feminine features is said to be a *male pseudohermaphrodite*—the child would have turned out to be a normal male if testosterone had been working properly during fetal life.

In this chapter we will review the various steps of sexual development to see how it is that things can go wrong—how girls turn into boys at puberty, why boys look like girls and girls like boys, and why occasionally it is difficult to tell which is what.

Genetic and Gonadal Sex Determination

Human chromosomes are very long strands of DNA surrounded by proteins and located inside the nuclei of cells. Each parent contributes 23 chromosomes; in each human cell there are 46 chromosomes, or 23 pairs. The pairs are numbered 1 to 22, and the sex chromosomes pair off either as XX or XY to make 23. Genetic regions (called genes) on the X and Y chromosomes are responsible, among other things, for the sexual orientation of the embryo during fetal life. The genetic program in the DNA of the sex chromosomes determines whether the gonads develop as ovaries or testes.

When a Y chromosome is present, the DNA of the Y chromosome directs the synthesis of proteins responsible for male development. One of these proteins, the so-called *H-Y antigen*, is located on the surface of cells in males of all mammalian species studied so far, whereas it is absent from female cells. The H-Y antigen may in fact be responsible for the original differentiation of the male testes in that early phase of embryonic life when primordial germ cells, after an arduous migration from the yolk sac across the dorsal mesentery to the gonadal ridge—like a west ridge Everest ascent—are preparing for their sexual assignment. Here, on the embryonic gonadal ridges, the primordial gonads are formed—indifferent gonads that look the same in male and female embryos, gonads poised to go either way, boy or girl, depending on the genetic instructions and the H-Y antigen.

The discovery of the H-Y antigen occurred unexpectedly—as is often the case in scientific research—during the investigation of a completely unrelated problem. Researchers noted in 1955 that female mice rejected skin grafts from identical inbred male mice, which means that the females developed antibodies against an antigen on the surface of male cells. This antigen (a substance that reacts with antibodies) was then named the Y-linked histocompatibility antigen or H-Y antigen.

The Y chromosome appears to be dominant in human sexual differentiation. When it is present, testes arise in the embryo and a male phenotype results; when it is absent, ovaries arise and a female phenotype results. Occasionally things go wrong. The genotype 47, XXY (47 chromosomes with an extra X chromosome) results in a male with *Klinefelter's syndrome*, an unusual syndrome characterized by normal-appearing male genitalia with small malfunctioning testes incapable of making spermatozoa. A rather common disorder, it occurs in about one of every 500 male births. Similarly, the genotypes XXXY, XXXXY, XYY, and XXYY are all phenotypic males, clearly indicating that the presence of a single Y chromosome confers maleness, possibly through the H-Y antigen, since all of the genotypes from XY to XXXXY have H-Y antigen present on the surface of their cells.

Conversely, the genotypes 46, XX (normal female), 47, XXX and 45, X0 (0 indicates no extra X chromosome and no Y chromosome) result in phenotypic females. The 45, X0 genotype is probably the most common genetic anomaly, occurring in about one of every 125 conceptions; but only about 3 percent of these 45, X0 embryos survive to birth. This means an incidence of one in 10,000 newborn females have the condition called *Turner's syndrome*, characterized by short stature, various skeletal anomalies, and nonfunctioning fibrotic ovaries. These patients often come to medical attention because they fail to menstruate and show no breast development at the time of puberty—all of which illustrates the importance of the second X chromosome in normal female development. The ovaries of aborted 45, X0 fetuses are perfectly normal, and yet at birth these babies with Turner's syndrome have streaked ovaries. Without the presence of the second X chromosome, the ovaries deteriorate during uterine life and yield streaks of fibrous tissue by the time of birth. None of the female genotypes XX, XXX, or X0 have detectable H-Y antigens on the surface of their cells, providing further evidence that the synthesis of this antigen is somehow directed by the Y chromosome. The 45, Y0 genotype does not exist in living humans, indicating that the absence of an X chromosome, in contrast to the Y chromosome, is incompatible with life.

The rule that the 46, XY genotype gives rise to H-Y antigen-positive males with normal testes, and the 46, XX genotype produces H-Y antigen-negative females with normal ovaries holds true most of the time. There are, however, some rather disconcerting exceptions to this simple view of sexual differentiation. Rare cases of normal males with well developed testes and a 46, XX genotype have been described. H-Y antigen is present in these cases, indicating that the region of the missing Y chromosome that regulates H-Y antigen and the formation of testes has been translocated to another chromosome.

Similarly, most true hermaphrodites have the 46, XX female genotype, and yet the testicular tissue present is positive and the ovarian tissue negative for the H-Y antigen, suggesting that some complex shuffling of genetic elements has occurred in these persons. To add more turbulence to an already complicated situation, there exist 46, XY females with streaked ovaries who may be either H-Y antigen-negative or positive. These rare cases point out that the presence of a Y chromosome or of H-Y antigen is not the whole story in the regulation of the transformation of indifferent gonads into testes. The whole story awaits further research, but in the meantime there is no reason for panic. In the vast majority of cases the 46, XY genotype leads to normal male development and the 46, XX genotype leads to normal female development, insuring that the species will shuffle along on its present path of astounding diversity.

Hormonal Regulation of Sexual Differentiation

We have seen, then, that genetic (chromosomal) sex is determined at the time of fertilization, when the die is cast in the female or male direction by chromosomal pairings of 46, XX or 46, XY. The next step is the formation of testes or ovaries. This is directed by a genetic blueprint in which the Y chromosome, through the H-Y antigen genes (and possibly other factors), directs the formation of testes; the absence of the H-Y antigen results in the formation of ovaries. Everything else that happens in sexual development is governed by the presence of these gonads.

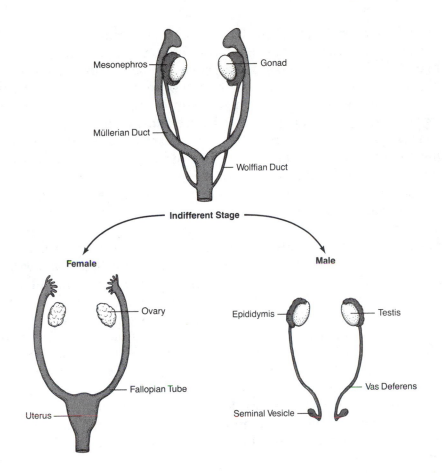

Figure 6-1. The indifferent müllerian and wolffian ducts transform into female and male internal genitalia during fetal development.

The details of this remarkable process were elaborated by the research of Alfred Jost in France during the late 1940s. Jost was interested in just how the gonads control development of the internal and external genitalia in mammals. Early in the embryonic life of mammalian fetuses the male and female internal genitalia appear as identical undifferentiated structures, each composed of wolffian and müllerian ducts; they differentiate later (see Figure 6-1) into male and female structures. In the male (XY) fetus the müllerian ducts regress and the wolffian ducts become the male internal genitalia.

Just the opposite events occur in female (XX) fetuses; the wolffian ducts regress and the female internal genitalia are formed from the müllerian ducts. Jost began by removing the gonads from female rabbits before sexual differentiation occurred and discovered, surprisingly, that the fetus developed into a normal female despite the absence of gonads. He concluded that castration of early female embryos has no effect on fetal sex development. With or without the ovaries the female fetus will undergo normal development, implying that the ovaries play no role in promoting female sexual differentiation, that they're just sitting around at this point, waiting to play an important role later on at the time of puberty.

Jost's most surprising finding was that if the gonads are removed from a male rabbit embryo, then the fetus will develop into a female. The time of castration is critical to the outcome of the experiment; it must occur early enough to prevent masculinization of the fetus by the testes. In rabbit fetuses, testes can be distinguished from ovaries by day 15 of the pregnancy, but the genitalia are identical until after day 20, and by day 26 sexual differentiation is well under way. If the rabbit fetus is castrated on day 19 or before, the fetus will develop into a normal female; castration after day 25 results in a normal male. These castration experiments in rabbits led Jost to the conclusion that fetal testes secrete hormones designed to regulate two processes—the formation of male genitalia, and the regression of the müllerian ducts, which would otherwise become female internal genitalia.

The import of the Jost experiments is that castrated mammalian fetuses of either chromosomal sex will develop as females—*that nature tends toward the female unless there is active intervention by hormones secreted from fetal testes to shift development to the male direction.* This leads to the Jost theory of sexual development, which can be viewed as the central dogma of this field: "Chromosomal sex determines gonadal sex; when the gonads are ovaries, or when no gonads are present, the fetus develops into a female phenotype; when the gonads are testes, then specific hormone secretions are elaborated which direct fetal sexual development into a male phenotype." Jost was able to deduce from further experiments that the two testicular secretions responsible for regulation of male development were an androgen and a müllerian regression factor, subsequently shown by others to be what is called testosterone, and the peptide hormone called müllerian regression hormone. This work has been extended to humans, particularly by Jean Wilson and his colleagues at the University of Texas Southwestern Medical School.

Normal female development in the human (illustrated schematically in Figure 6-2) following germ cell migration to the genital ridge shows that little differentiation occurs until about the ninth week of gestation. Then development of internal genitalia begins, followed by wolffian duct degeneration and external genitalia development—all during the first trimester. In the second trimester, ovarian follicles containing eggs mature, while the synthesis of estradiol by the ovary declines. This pattern of normal female development occurs in the presence of ovaries; but in the absence of ovaries or testes a similar pattern will occur. Starting at two months of gestation the female hormone, estradiol, is produced by the ovaries. Its function, however, is not known, since in the absence of ovaries, and consequently in the absence of estradiol, the fetus still undergoes normal female development. (The ovaries play an important role at puberty, at which time estradiol leads to female sexual characteristics and follicle maturation leads to fertility.)

Male sexual development during fetal life plays out along entirely different lines (see Figure 6-3). Here the male testes begin to synthesize müllerian regression hormone and testosterone at about eight weeks of gestation. This leads to early regression of the müllerian ducts (which would have developed into fallopian tubes and a uterus in the absence of müllerian regression hormone). Testosterone produced by the Leydig cells in the fetal testes stimulates wolffian duct differentiation into the vas deferens and seminal vesicles; thus testosterone transforms the wolffian ducts into male internal genitalia. Actually, testosterone itself does not transform the external genitalia into male structures; this is accomplished by a derivative of testosterone called dihydrotestosterone (DHT), produced from testosterone by an enzyme inside those cells destined to differentiate into the male scrotum and penis. When there is a deficiency of the enzyme, ambiguous genitalia result at birth. The baby may appear to be female and then later at puberty turn into a male, as did the children in the Dominican Republic.

Females with Masculine Characteristics

The vast majority of fetuses with a 46, XX female chromosomal sex develop a normal female gonadal sex with bilateral ovaries and will have normal female internal and external genitalia. Not much can go wrong here since, as we have seen, testes are normally necessary to masculinize a fetus and to promote müllerian duct regression. However, Murphy's Law still applies—if things can go wrong they will—

FEMALE DEVELOPMENT

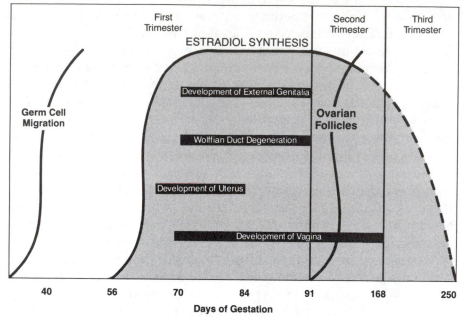

Figure 6-2. The normal sequence of sexual development during fetal life of the human female

MALE DEVELOPMENT

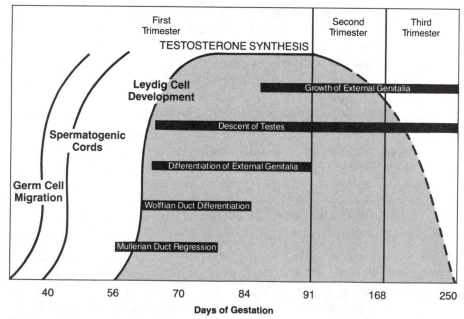

Figure 6-3. The normal sequence of sexual development during fetal life of the human male

and in this situation they occasionally do: Girls can turn out to look like boys, and when they do they are called *female pseudohermaphrodites*—a long term to describe children with female genetic and gonadal sex, but who, in addition, have some masculine features of the external genitalia.

Female pseudohermaphrodites all result from the same basic problem, the exposure of a female fetus to excess androgens (male hormones) in embryonic life—before 12 weeks of gestation. After 12 weeks androgens will cause enlargement of the clitoris but no other structural abnormalities. Before 12 weeks, however, exposure of a female fetus to androgens can lead to severe masculinization of the external genitalia. One source of excess androgens can be the mother, who may take androgenlike pills or injections, or may have an androgen-secreting tumor of the ovaries or adrenal gland. Any excessive androgens in the maternal circulation can be transmitted to the fetus and cause male differentiation of the external genitalia. Occasionally a female fetus will produce its own excess androgens from the adrenal glands. (This happens when the synthesis of cortisol from cholesterol in the adrenal glands is blocked by faulty enzymes in the synthetic chain of chemical reactions. The pituitary reacts to falling blood levels of cortisol by producing ACTH, which stimulates the adrenal gland to make more cortisol. In doing this the adrenal gland also synthesizes more androgens.)

Fortunately, the exposure of female fetuses to androgens is uncommon, and when it does occur the children can be treated to prevent further excess androgen production, and plastic surgery repair of the external genitalia can be accomplished. The internal genitalia, including the uterus and fallopian tubes, are normally unaffected, as no müllerian regression hormone is present because there are no testes, and the excessive androgen levels do not affect the müllerian structures.

Males with Feminine Characteristics

Normal human male sexual differentiation during fetal development requires that a number of intricate metabolic steps work harmoniously to bend nature away from its natural predilection toward femaleness. While little can go wrong in female fetal sexual development to lead to a masculinized fetus, there are all kinds of opportunities for error in male sexual development that can lead to feminization of the fetus. To avoid this, several tasks must be accomplished: the fetal testes must synthesize müllerian regression hormone and testosterone properly, and these hormones must then interact with receptors at the target cells. Receptors must be present and capable of converting the hormone signal into an effective intracellular message. Tissues destined to become male external genitalia must have a normally functioning enzyme (called 5α-reductase) capable of converting the precursor hormone testosterone into the active hormone dihydrotestosterone (DHT). Finally, the intracellular machinery responsible for translating the hormone-receptor interaction message must be intact. Children with the male chromosomal sex 46, XY and testes for gonads, but who are nevertheless feminized by errors in sexual differentiation, are called male pseudohermaphrodites because they are male in genetic and gonadal sex but have physical features that are female in appearance.

The most common underlying cause of male pseudohermaphroditism, responsible for about 75 percent of the cases, is some form of resistance to testosterone; that is, the hormone doesn't work normally at its target cells even though a normal or even elevated amount is circulating in the blood. The syndromes of androgen resistance (failure to connect at the target) come in many shapes and sizes, but generally they can be classified into three basic types of defect (see Figure 6-4). The intracellular androgen receptor depicted by the symbol R can be defective to a variable degree and thereby give rise to a considerable range of clinical abnormalities; the enzyme that converts testosterone to DHT can be defective, or the interaction of the hormone-receptor complex with DNA in the nucleus may be abnormal. These three different mechanisms of androgen resistance lead to a tremendous diversity of clinical disorders.

Early in the nineteenth century the first patients with testicular feminization began to be reported in the medical literature, and since then a large number of cases have been recognized. This disorder occurs in 46, XY genetic males who are completely resistant to the action of testosterone and dihydrotestosterone because of an abnormality of the male hormone receptor. Since testosterone doesn't work in these patients, the wolffian ducts regress to leave no male internal genitalia. DHT doesn't work either, so the external genitalia are female without ambiguity. Müllerian regression hormone is produced by the testes and it functions normally, so that the müllerian ducts regress, leaving no female internal genitalia.

Patients with the testicular feminization syndrome are born and raised as normal-appearing females but with testes sequestered in the abdomen or the inguinal canal. At puberty they develop into normal females except that they have no menstrual bleeding. A medical work-up at this time, if it includes an abdominal exploration, reveals that they have testes (which are removed surgically because of a tendency to undergo malignant transformation), but no uterus or fallopian tubes—and no male internal genitalia either. Blood levels of testosterone are high, often above the normal male levels, and the blood level of the pituitary hormone LH is elevated (because the pituitary cells that make LH also have abnormal androgen receptors and therefore do not respond to feedback inhibition by the elevated serum testosterone level). Since hair on the face, under the arms, and in the pubic area requires androgen stimulation to grow, hair is missing from these regions in patients with testicular feminization.

This syndrome is not uncommon; it is the third leading cause of the failure of girls to menstruate at puberty. A number of famous women, among them a movie star, have had the testicular feminization syndrome; they obviously can and do lead normal lives as women except that they are not able to have children. Even though they start out at fertilization to be 46, XY males with the formation of normal testes, they turn out to be well-developed females because the testosterone produced by the testes and its metabolite DHT do not work on their target cells. These individuals are able to go through puberty and develop normal female contours because the testosterone produced by the testes is converted to a potent estrogen (estradiol) in the liver and other tissues. In the testicular feminization syndrome the binding of testosterone and DHT to androgen receptors in target tissues is defective, although the conversion of testosterone to estradiol is normal—as is the action of estradiol with estrogen receptors—allowing the female secondary sexual characteristics to develop on schedule. This syndrome certainly illustrates that nature tends to the female—boys turn into girls when the male hormones don't work.

When androgen receptor defects are less severe, some masculinization of the fetus occurs along with some feminization, so that ambiguity in sex assignment may arise. These partial defects in androgen receptors give rise to a broad array of clinical disorders, ranging from infertility in normal-appearing males to small vaginal pouches and female breast development. These syndromes, like the testicular feminization syndrome, are characterized by high serum levels of LH and testosterone and increased estrogen production, indicating the presence of resistance to androgens. Where one stands, then, on the line

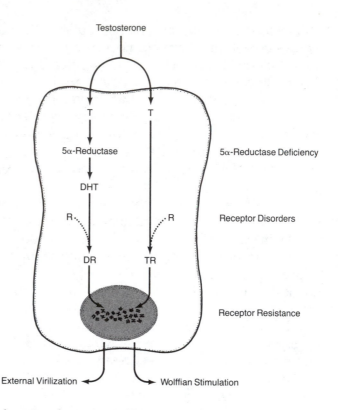

Figure 6-4. Resistance to the action of testosterone (T) can occur at three different sites inside of target cells. The androgen receptor (R) binds with T or its metabolite DHT (dihydrotestosterone) in the cell cytoplasm and the bound complex then enters the cell nucleus where it exerts its action.

between a normal-appearing male and a normal-appearing female depends on the degree of abnormality of the androgen receptor.

In the early 1960s, case reports of a unique androgen resistance syndrome began to be reported: Children with ambiguous genitalia who were raised as girls became severely masculinized at puberty. In 1974, Wilson described two of these patients from Dallas and Imperato-McGinley described 24 from the Dominican Republic. Both research groups demonstrated that the basic problem was a deficiency of the *5α-reductase* enzyme that converts testosterone to dihydrotestosterone (DHT). Eventually a total of 38 patients with this disorder were discovered in the Dominican Republic. The scientific importance of this syndrome lies in its elucidation of the role of DHT in sexual differentiation. These patients are 46, XY genetic males with testes that produce normal amounts of testosterone and müllerian regression hormone; thus they have normal male internal genitalia and no female internal structures. And yet they appear feminine at birth because they lack the normal levels of DHT required to masculinize the external genitalia. When things go wrong with the production of DHT the external genitalia become feminine during fetal life. At puberty the testes produce an increased amount of testosterone, and more DHT is produced, even though the 5α-reductase enzyme is not functioning normally. This results in a male-appearing teen-ager who has been transformed from a girl to a boy with male external genitalia—a fate that most of these patients seem able to accept.

Resistance to the action of testosterone or DHT is not the only cause of male pseudohermaphroditism. Any disorder that leads to a decrease in the synthesis of testosterone by Leydig cells in the testes will obviously cause trouble. About 25 percent of the cases of male pseudohermaphrodites result from enzyme defects in the biosynthetic pathway that leads to the synthesis of testosterone from cholesterol. There are about six enzymatic steps between cholesterol and testosterone, and each of these enzymes can be rendered defective by genetic mutations in the DNA segment that codes for the enzyme. Children with such enzyme defects are 46, XY genetic males with testes who, like the children with the more common androgen resistance syndromes, have ambiguous external genitalia. Occasionally the Leydig cells fail to develop normally, yielding 46, XY patients with a nearly normal female appearance. Patients with poorly developed Leydig cells or defects in the biosynthesis of testosterone can be easily distinguished from patients with one of the androgen resistance syndromes, because the former will have low serum testosterone levels compared to the latter group.

Finally, there is a rare group of genetic 46, XY males who fail to make müllerian regression hormone but who have no abnormalities in testosterone synthesis or action. As one would predict from the above analysis, these patients develop as normal-appearing males, thanks to the presence of testosterone and DHT in normal quantities and their normal interaction with androgen receptors. However, because müllerian regression hormone is not present, they end up with a uterus and with fallopian tubes in addition to the normal male internal genitalia. This is fortunately a very rare disorder.

As we have seen, male sexual differentiation is complex, requiring a number of intricate steps to be intact. Any mistake in the cascade allows nature to drift into its natural feminine course and leads to the feminization of the genetic 46, XY male fetus. The degree of feminization depends on the type and severity of the defect in synthesis or action of müllerian regression hormone, testosterone, or dihydrotestosterone, the hormonal triumvirate whose coordinated action is essential for normal male sexual development.

Hormone Regulation of Sexual Behavior

One glance at the genitalia of the newborn child usually tells the story—the gender is immediately apparent. This is a reasonable approach to sorting out if it's a girl or if it's a boy; occasionally, however, there is ambiguity. In the presence of ambiguous genitalia a more careful assessment is necessary to determine the proper gender assignment, a determination that will obviously have a lifelong impact on the child. Hormones play a central role in sexual differentiation of the fetus at the level of internal and external genitalia. We have seen that when these hormones are absent or not working properly, fetal development shifts in the female direction, irrespective of the genetic or gonadal sex of the embryo. At a critical point in embryonic life androgens impose a male imprint on the fetus, an imprint that consists of male external genitalia.

Do the high androgen levels seen in the fetus also imprint male characteristics other than the genitalia? Is there a male central nervous system that results from fetal androgens or a female counterpart that results from fetal estrogens? These questions are as yet unanswered for humans, but in other mammals it is quite clear that exposure of the animal to androgens early in life can permanently alter brain physiology in the male direction and change the innate animal reproductive behavior to male behavior.

Most adult female mammals have a cyclic pattern of ovulation (for example, 5 days in rats, 15 days in guinea pigs, 28 days in humans) which, as we have seen, results from the cyclic release of LH and FSH from the pituitary gland and its regulation by estradiol released from the ovaries. (The cyclic release of LH and FSH undoubtedly results from the cyclic release of LHRH from the hypothalamus.) Adult male mammals, on the other hand, show no such dramatic cyclic release of LH and FSH from their pituitary glands but rather demonstrate a monotonous episodic pattern of release every few hours. This male pattern of LH and FSH fluctuations also occurs in females, in addition to the monthly cyclic patten.

Geoffrey Harris, who developed the theory of hypothalamic hormone regulation of the pituitary, demonstrated that if a newborn male rat is castrated within 72 hours of birth, its brain is irreversibly feminized, so that at puberty the male rat will exhibit the female pattern of cyclic LH and FSH production. An ovary transplanted into such a castrated male rat after puberty will undergo cyclic ovulation just as it would in a female rat. Conversely, if the castrated newborn male rat is given a single injection of testosterone just after castration, no female cyclic gonadotropin pattern occurs in adulthood and a transplanted ovary will not ovulate. Similarly, if a newborn female rat is given an injection of testosterone just after birth, it will not ovulate as an adult but rather will show the male pattern of monotonous gonadotropin secretion.

Certain characteristic sexual behaviors in male and female rats are employed to promote reproduction. The female pattern involves cyclic periods of sexual receptivity timed with ovulation, whereas the male continually demonstrates certain mounting behaviors. It is clear that the presence of an androgen like testosterone in early life is critical for adult male sexual behavior, while its absence is essential for female behavior.

It is now apparent that testosterone can imprint maleness on the rat brain in a specific physiologic sense, and that in its absence the brain differentiates in a female direction. One of the surprising twists of fate in this story is that inside the brain cells testosterone is converted to the female hormone estradiol, and it is apparently the *estradiol* that masculinizes the brain. Estradiol receptors are located in specific regions of the brain, where the development and eventual function of neurons is presumably influenced directly by estradiol and indirectly by testosterone through its conversion to estradiol.

The exact regions of the brain where steroid sex hormones imprint their control on the brain physiology of lower mammals are not yet known, but several types of control seem to be involved. First is the imprinting of maleness by testosterone at an early stage when there is a presumed influence on the growth and development of specific neurons in the brain that relate to male or female reproductive functions. Later, the androgen and estrogen hormones appear important in promoting the physical changes of puberty as well as the behavioral components of maleness and femaleness.

It is not clear at present how the experimental findings in rats and other lower mammals relate to the regulation of human sexuality. No imprinting of the human brain by androgens or estrogens has been convincingly demonstrated to date. The hypothalamic-pituitary control of LH and FSH secretion can be switched from the tonic male pattern in adult male humans to the cyclic female pattern by exposing the males to cyclic administration of ovarian hormones, so that there appears to be no innate maleness in the human hypothalamus or pituitary regarding the regulation of the gonads. There is a condition in humans, called congenital adrenal hyperplasia (CAH), in which the adrenal gland makes an excess of androgen hormone (because of a defective enzyme in the synthetic pathway of cortisol). Girls born with this disorder have been exposed to an excess of androgens during fetal life and thus have masculinized external genitalia. When discovered early the condition can be treated by surgical correction of the external genitalia to a female appearance, and the excessive androgen production by the adrenals can be easily checked. During childhood these girls with CAH undergo normal female puberty, develop normal menstrual cycles, and show normal fertility. There seems to be no imprinting of maleness by exposure to excessive androgens during fetal life even though the external genitalia are masculinized. Girls who are exposed to androgen drugs by their mothers during fetal life also show no male imprinting, and after corrective genital surgery at birth develop as females capable of having their own children. There seems to be no impact on the child's ultimate psychosocial development as a normal woman. In this regard humans are strikingly different from lower mammals.

The view that cultural and psychiatric factors play the dominant role in human sexuality, with only minor hormonal contributions, was rolling along more or less uncontested until girls started turning into boys in the Dominican Republic. Of the 38 subjects with the guevedoce syndrome, 18 had been raised as girls, had gone through puberty, and were available for detailed interviewing. That nearly all of these 18 girls had transformed into boys during puberty without regret or great difficulty led Imperato-McGinley to the conclusion that androgens make a strong contribution to the formation of male gender identity, a contribution that can apparently override the psychosocial impact of being reared as a girl.

The villages studied by Imperato-McGinley are composed mostly of two-room, thatched-roof huts constructed of sticks. Villagers bathe primarily in the river, as very few huts have shower facilities. The villages are organized along strongly paternalistic lines, with double standards favoring sexual and other freedoms for men. Boys and girls are raised along very different paths, with a rather sharp distinction between male and female roles. The girls and boys play together until they are segregated at about age six or seven into separate male and female activities. The boys help their fathers with farming activities and generally have a considerable amount of freedom to play; they usually do not attend school. At about 12 years of age they begin going to bars and cockfights, and at 14 they begin visiting prostitutes (who are accepted as a fact of life). Boys usually marry between 18 and 25 years of age and settle down to a life of farming, mining, or chopping down trees for fuel. The girls are more confined; they spend most of their time around the home helping their mothers with household chores and usually marry between 13 and 20 years of age. Strict fidelity is demanded from them but not from the husbands.

Detailed interviews with the 18 affected subjects, as well as with their siblings, parents, neighbors, and girlfriends, revealed that all 18 had been unambiguously reared as girls. Thus, before puberty each had a female gender identity (subjective self-awareness of being female) and a female gender role (public expression by speech and actions of the female gender identity). In 17 of the 18 the gender identity gradually changed over several years, beginning before 12 years of age, as they began to feel and look like men. In 16 of the subjects there eventually occurred a switch to a male gender role at an average age of 16, and 15 of these subjects eventually lived with a woman. These males are able to have sexual intercourse but they have not fathered children.

Between fetal life and puberty (when the pituitary gonadotropins and gonadal steroids are at a high level) there is a long dormant period of about ten years when the hypothalamic-pituitary-gonadal axis is shut down in a resting phase waiting to spring to life at the onset of puberty. Puberty is heralded by small nocturnal pulsations of LH, undoubtedly resulting from nocturnal pulsations of LHRH from the hypothalamus. Why the hypothalamus remains dormant for ten years and then suddenly begins to give forth little nighttime blips of LHRH is a mystery related to maturation of the brain. However, once the LHRH starts to pulse, the floodgates are open, as this initiates pituitary release of LH and FSH, which in turn stimulate the testes to produce testosterone and sperm and the ovaries to produce estradiol and eggs. The nocturnal LHRH pulsations gradually give way to round-the-clock pulsations occurring episodically at intervals of several hours. Eventually in females a monthly cyclic pattern of LH and FSH is integrated with ovulation and estradiol secretion from the ovaries.

Profound transformations are directed by hormones during fetal life and again at puberty to shape our sexual destiny. The embryo tends toward the female unless androgens and müllerian regression factor from testes intervene to bend the natural tendency toward male differentiation. This is a complex process, and if anything goes wrong with the androgens then feminization will result. After a long dormant phase of about ten years the hormones return again to fire up the transformations of puberty and preserve the secondary sexual characteristics of adult life. Without these hormones reproductive life would be impossible and the species would grind to a halt, strangled by a fatal loss of sexuality and fertility.

7

GIANTS AND DWARFS

■

There is not much you can do to become tall if you have inherited genes that say you are supposed to be short; there are, however, plenty of ways to end up short even if you are genetically programmed to be tall. This is because maximum growth requires an optimal balance of nutrition and hormones. When food is in short supply, as it unfortunately is in many parts of the world, then the skeleton and other body organ systems don't grow at an optimal rate; growth is stunted if the scarce nutrients needed to supply the body's basic energy requirements are not available. Thyroid hormone and growth hormone are both essential for normal growth. Any disorder that limits the supply of either in early life will also result in stunting. Chronic infections and malignancies can decrease growth, as can emotional deprivation.

Good health, good nutrition, and the normal functioning of thyroid hormone and growth hormone are all required for the achievement of maximal adult height. Given good health and nutrition, the most important regulator is growth hormone, which will be our focus in this chapter. Giants and dwarfs result from the abnormal action of growth hormone—giants from an excess of growth hormone beginning in early life, and dwarfs from either a deficiency or an inactivity of growth hormone.

Gigantism

Robert Wadlow was born in Alton, Illinois, in the year 1928. At birth he weighed 8½ pounds and was normal in height; there was no clue in his modest beginning to suggest that he would soon become known as "the Alton giant" and eventually grow to a height of 8 feet 11 inches,

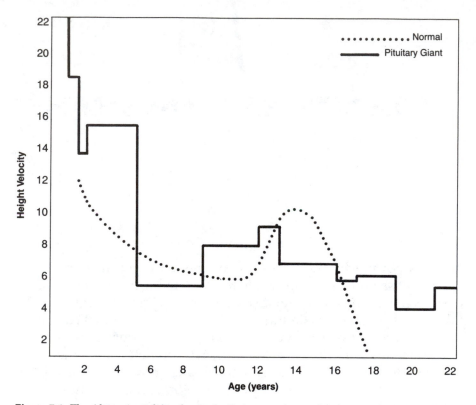

Figure 7-1. The Alton giant showed a markedly increased growth velocity in early life and then a steady growth velocity after five years of age. Note the difference between the growth velocity of the Alton giant and that of a normal person.

the tallest human being ever recorded in a verifiable fashion. Shortly after birth he began to grow at an acceleration so rapid that by one year of age he weighed 62 pounds and was about 3 feet 8 inches tall (see Figure 7-1). He grew very rapidly in the early years of his life and never stopped growing. By the time he was 9, he weighed 178 pounds and had grown to a height of 6 feet 1 inch. This remarkable growth pattern continued unabated until his death from infection at 22 years of age, when he weighed 475 pounds and measured 107 inches in height.

Skull x-rays show that he had a pituitary tumor, undoubtedly the culprit: First, the tumor produced excessive amounts of growth hormone starting at an early age, so that his growth rate got off to a flying start. Second, the tumor compressed neighboring pituitary tissue, hampering production of the gonadotropins LH and FSH and result-

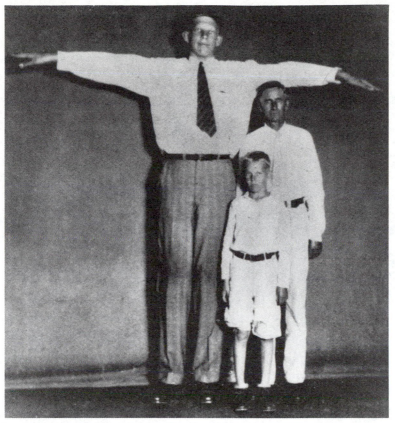

The Alton giant Robert Wadlow developed a growth-hormone secreting pituitary tumor early in his life. At age 13 he already towered over his father and his nine-year old brother.

ing in deficient testosterone production by the testes. Because he lacked the blood level of testosterone necessary for normal bone maturation, the growth plates at the ends of the long bones of the Alton giant remained immature and continued to grow throughout his life. He grew to be the tallest human on record because the tumor became active so early in his life, probably shortly after his birth. Later in his short life the Alton giant was severely incapacitated by damage to the nerves in his extremities, so that he had recurrent foot infections. Gigantism generally results in a shortened life span and these infections caused his death at the young age of 22 years. It is unlikely that this will ever happen again, at least in industrialized societies, because we can now diagnose and treat gigantism before it becomes so far advanced.

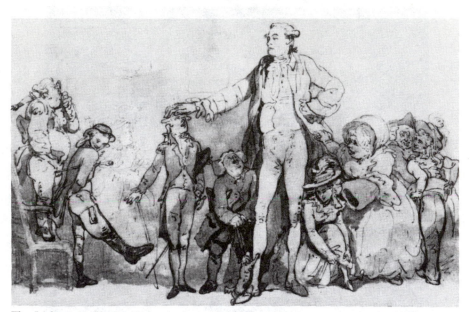

The Irish giant Charles Byrne is depicted in comparison to friends in a 1785 drawing by Rowlandson.

When these same tumors arise after puberty, at a time when the growth plates have matured and the bones have stopped growing, a different type of syndrome occurs. The bones and soft tissues thicken but do not lengthen, producing the condition called *acromegaly*. Thus, gigantism and acromegaly are two different manifestations of the same problem, namely, the appearance in the pituitary gland of a growth-hormone-secreting tumor. Acromegaly only rarely results from a tumor that secretes growth-hormone-releasing hormone (GHRH), but it is from several of these tumors that the structure of GHRH has been identified.

Throughout history giants have held great fascination for many, even though they are exceedingly rare and not of great clinical importance. Most people—and most physicians—will live their entire lives without ever seeing a real giant. Bruno Bettelheim emphasizes that the giants in fairy tales symbolize adults who can often be outwitted by cunning children. Adults appear like selfish giants to children, and, whether we like it or not, children delight in the idea that we are easy to fool. Giants abound in Nordic mythology, and Biblical references to giants are scattered throughout the Old Testament, culminating in the story of the Philistine Goliath of Gath, whose height was

6 cubits and a span (over 9 feet tall). Although it is possible that Goliath had a growth-hormone-producing pituitary tumor, it is difficult to believe that he could be afflicted with gigantism and still possess great physical strength. The Greek historian Herodotus described a man named Artachnaeos who was about 8 feet 2 inches tall and supposedly had the loudest voice in the world. It is interesting that patients with acromegaly characteristically have deep husky voices.

The famous Irish giants Cornelius Magrath and Charles Byrne, like the Alton giant, died in their early 20s. Byrne was born in Ireland in 1761 and as a child grew rapidly to a huge size—a phenomenon that was attributed to his conception on top of a haystack! During his teenage years he was displayed at local fairs, and at 21 he was exhibited in London, where it was claimed that at 8 feet 2 inches he was the tallest man in the world. His alcoholic excesses led to his death the following year, and on his deathbed he requested that his body be thrown into the sea to keep his bones away from the fraternity of surgeons who were lusting after his skeleton. This was obviously not enough to keep the surgeons at bay, as can be seen in the photograph which shows the gigantic skeleton of Charles Byrne residing in the John Hunter Museum in England. No one knows exactly how the famous English surgeon Hunter acquired the skeleton; however, an unverified account has it that he bribed the undertakers to allow the Byrne skeleton to be included in his collection of some 13,000 biological specimens now in the John Hunter Museum presently maintained by the Royal College of Surgeons.

Entry into the Hunter collection of biological specimens was only a starting point in a long sequence of scientific studies of the Byrne skeleton that has continued to the present day. At the time the skeleton was diverted from the ocean to the Hunter collection in 1783, the theory that the pituitary was a clearing house for brain waste products secreted as a nasal discharge still prevailed. There was no way for anyone to know that the Irish giant had a large pituitary tumor sitting in an enlarged and eroded sella turcica. Following the discovery of acromegaly by Pierre Marie in 1886 and subsequent proposals that both gigantism and acromegaly might be caused by pituitary tumors, Arthur Keith, curator of the John Hunter Museum, and Harvey Cushing, a prominent American neurosurgeon, opened the Byrne skull in 1909. They found a grossly enlarged sella turcica that had undoubtedly resulted from a pituitary tumor. Hunter had missed his chance to connect gigantism to pituitary tumors. In 1963 skull x-rays of the

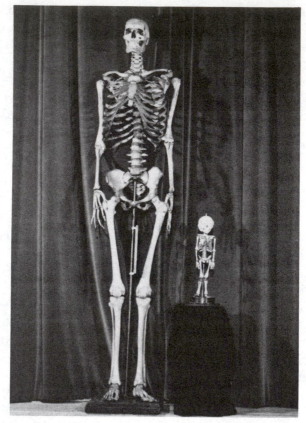

The skeleton of the Irish giant Charles Byrne now hangs in the John Hunter Museum alongside the skeleton of the Sicilian dwarf.

Byrne skeleton showed bone changes consistent with a pituitary tumor and acromegaly. Finally, wrist x-rays of the skeleton in 1980 revealed that Byrne, like the Alton giant, had pituitary insufficiency and did not make enough testoserone to close the growth plates at the end of the forearm bone.

It's no fun being a giant. Excessive amounts of growth hormones— and other growth factors called somatomedins—are constantly circulating around with detrimental effects on the body. At the same time, a growth-hormone-producing tumor may be causing the pituitary to secrete *too little* of other hormones. Gigantism and acromegaly both result from the excessive secretion of growth hormone by the pituitary gland, and at the present time they are treatable disorders with the potential for a cure. Gigantism occurs when bones are exposed to the consequences of excessive growth hormone while they are still able to grow, before the bone growth plates have closed. Acromegaly occurs after bones are no longer capable of growing; so the body thickens and distorts but does not lengthen. Giants who live long enough will develop some features of acromegaly; after a long period of lengthening, their bodies will begin to thicken. The life of a giant in real life and in fairy tales is often one of misery and early death—not the kind of life, even if you happen to be short, that you should wish for.

Dwarfs and Pygmies

Dwarfs, like giants, are objects of intense interest in many human societies and occupy a prominent place in fairy tales and folklore. Often stunted in emotional as well as physical growth, they are fixed in a pre-sexual phase of life, devoted to hard work and the acquisition of material goods. Satisfied with their unchanging daily existence of toil and lack of intimate relationships, they are workers of the earth who boil life down to a meat and potatoes basis. They can be very nasty but they can also be extremely benevolent, rescuing your daughter in the woods in time to save her from the sadistic excesses of your second wife.

Real dwarfs are stunted primarily in physical growth, a condition often effectively treated with preparations of human growth hormone. The growth of bones and other tissues is a complex metabolic process, and, as one might imagine, many steps of this process can go wrong. On a worldwide basis the most common causes of diminished growth in children are malnutrition and chronic disease. Short stature can also result from intrinsic defects in bone growth as a result of genetic defects, chromosomal abnormalities, congenital anomalies, and other ill-defined rare syndromes. Fortunately, these conditions are uncommon and are not generally encountered in the day-to-day practice of medicine.

The growth characteristics of humans are shown in Figure 7-2 as an idealized set of growth curves similar in shape to what one would see in other primates. The growth velocity curve is simply the first derivative of the growth curve and shows several interesting features about human growth characteristics. There is a steep decline in growth velocity during the first several years of life, which levels off after four years until puberty, when a growth spurt occurs. Finally, in the mid- to late teen-age years the growth velocity reaches zero, and height levels off for a while. Each of us shrinks a small amount over time, but

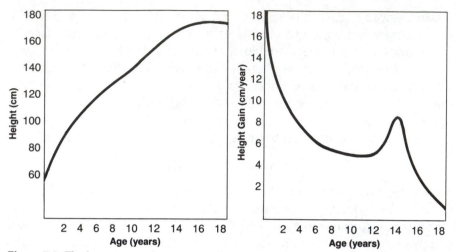

Figure 7-2. The human growth curve shows a rapid gain in height in early life and a growth spurt during puberty.

this is a result of the aging of bones and is not a process that is mediated by changes in growth hormone action. The growth profiles shown in Figure 7-2 are slightly different for each individual, limited by genetic programs that give rise to a whole range of growth velocities and growth curves. For a society, the normal range—defined as the heights for a given age that are between the third and ninety-seventh percentile—is dependent on race, sex, and environmental factors related to nutrition and prevailing chronic diseases. The dwarfs fall far below the third percentile and are often recognizable in early childhood.

Pituitary dwarfs result when the pituitary gland fails to produce an adequate amount of growth hormone, or when normally secreted growth hormone does not work properly at its target sites. The growth-regulating-hormone cascade starts in the hypothalamus with the cells producing growth-hormone-releasing hormone (GHRH) and somatostatin. Any process that leads to a deficiency of GHRH or an excess of somatostatin in the hypothalamus will result in a growth hormone deficiency. The most common cause of growth hormone deficiency in childhood is an ill-defined defect in hypothalamic regulation that may in some cases result from oxygen deprivation at birth. In rare instances, the hypothalamus fails to function normally in children who are exposed to an environment of severe psychosocial deprivation; growth returns when these children are removed to a better environment. Brain tumors, such as the dreaded craniopharyngioma, and inflammatory diseases involving the hypothalamus or pituitary gland can also lead to growth hormone deficiency. These disorders all produce pituitary dwarfism.

Dwarfism is often first noted when a child fails to follow a normal growth curve (see Figure 7-2). We can now treat many of these cases if they are discovered early enough. New neurosurgical techniques in removal of pituitary tumors have revolutionized the treatment of pituitary tumors, and growth hormone is now available to stimulate normal growth. Unlike the dwarfs of fairy tales, many of these young persons can now look forward to a more normal adult life.

A new type of dwarf was first described in 1966 by Zoi Laron and his colleagues in Israel. These so-called "Laron dwarfs" are from Jewish families of Asiatic origin and they look exactly like pituitary dwarfs with growth hormone deficiency. Actually, however, the Laron dwarfs have elevated blood levels of growth hormone and low levels of the growth factors called somatomedins; furthermore they fail to grow when they are treated with growth hormone—circulating growth hormone just does not work in these patients. Initially it was conjectured that the Laron dwarfs synthesized an aberrant growth hormone that showed up in the serum growth hormone assay but did not work at the target sites. More recent research, however, indicates that growth hormone circulating in the serum of Laron dwarfs is normal; the problem is that it doesn't work at its usual target sites, a phenomenon that can be described as resistance to growth hormone action. One of the sites is the liver, where growth hormone normally promotes the synthesis of the somatomedins.

Their low somatomedin levels may contribute to the growth retardation of Laron dwarfs. Their elevated growth hormone levels may be attributable to the lack of feedback regulation provided by normal levels of somatomedins on the pituitary cells that make growth hormone. When purified somatomedins become available in sufficient quantities, it will be interesting to see if they can promote growth in the Laron dwarfs, thus sparing these unfortunate children the disadvantages of their extremely small stature.

The pygmies of central Africa have long been of great interest to endocrinologists and others concerned with growth abnormalities. These fascinating dwarflike peoples may be among the oldest inhabitants of the African continent. Two pygmy tribes, the M'buti and the Babingas, are racially distinct from neighboring tribes. Over the past 20 years, Rimoin, Merimee, and their associates have made several expeditions to Central Africa to study the growth characteristics of the Babinga pygmies and have uncovered some interesting findings. The pygmies appear to have a defect in the production of one of the somatomedins called somatomedin C. The average height of a Babinga adult female is 4 feet 10 inches, while the males average 5 feet; their body proportions, measured as the ratio of the upper body length to the lower body length, are similar to the proportions of 6-year-old American Blacks. In their initial expeditions Rimoin and Merimee found that the pygmies had normal blood levels of growth hormone and that growth hormone was released normally from the pituitary gland. But growth hormone injected into the pygmies did not produce any effects, whereupon they concluded that pygmies are unresponsive to the effects of growth hormone.

Initial somatomedin measurements (recall that somatomedins are growth factors) in the pygmies indicated that the blood somatomedin levels were normal; however, as the assays have become more sophisticated and precise, it appears that these people may have a defect in the production of one of the important somatomedins. A recent study by Merimee and his colleagues shows that the pygmies do not have normal blood levels of somatomedin C, a possible explanation for their being so short. The value of all this research to the pygmies is not clear even if it turns out that their growth rate could be increased by somatomedin C. Perhaps they would just like to be pygmies and suspect that the scientists are trying to figure out a way for everyone else to become small like them.

In summary, then, abnormally short stature can result from defects in the synthesis of growth hormone by the pituitary gland (pituitary dwarfs), defects in the action of growth hormone (Laron dwarfs), defects in the production of somatomedins (pygmies), and possibly defects in the action of the somatomedins.

The Physiology of Growth Hormone

Real giants and dwarfs do exist and have been known since antiquity, but the idea that a substance exists whose presence in excess or whose absence could produce these rare disorders was slow in evolving and had little scientific support until the early 1920s, when Evans and Long grew giant rats by injecting normal rats with extracts prepared from the pituitary glands of cattle. These experiments proved beyond a doubt that the pituitary gland contains a growth-promoting substance; after several more decades of painstaking research this substance was finally isolated as growth hormone. The pituitary glands of cattle and other mammals contain a large amount of growth hormone, far more of it than any other hormone—a fortunate twist of fate that made it easier to isolate growth hormone and ultimately made possible successful treatment of patients with dwarfism.

It took many years to develop the chemical techniques necessary to isolate pure growth hormone from cattle and pigs. These were developed during the 1940s, a decade that also saw many studies demonstrating the effectiveness of growth hormone preparations in promoting growth in lower mammals. The investigators, however, were severely frustrated by the fact that none of the growth hormone preparations from cattle or pigs was effective in humans. A cure for human dwarfism was at hand, but the cure didn't work—and the reason was not at all apparent for many years. A new approach to the problem was needed and it came from an unexpected direction. In 1954 Wilhelmi and Pickford discovered that growth hormone prepared from fish was effective in fish, as expected, but was not active in rats—in other words, growth hormone appeared to be species specific. Shortly after this new insight broadened the thinking about growth hormone, Knobil and Greep found that growth hormone isolated from monkey pituitaries was active when injected into monkeys, but the growth hormone isolated from cattle and pigs did not become active if injected into monkeys.

Thus it became obvious that the structure of growth hormone varied from species to species and that the cure for human dwarfism would only arise from the isolation of human growth hormone. The first step was to develop a method for isolating growth hormone from human cadaver pituitaries, which was accomplished by Maury Raben at the New England Center Hospital in Boston in 1956. John Beck and his colleagues at the Royal Victoria Hospital in Montreal next demonstrated that the Raben hormone preparation promoted growth in a human dwarf whose deficiency had resulted from the absence of growth hormone. The National Pituitary Agency was established to collect human pituitary glands from all over North America, and for many years these pituitary gland collections have served as the sole source of growth hormone available to treat children with growth disorders. The determination of its chemical structure was accomplished in the early 1970s, and human growth hormone has now been synthesized by recombinant DNA techniques in bacteria. We now

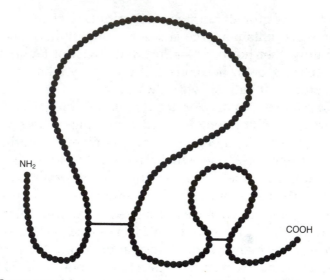

Figure 7-3. Human growth hormone contains 191 amino acids. There are two loops with disulfide bonds at their bases.

have a potentially unlimited source of growth hormone, which will undoubtedly eventually replace human cadaver pituitary glands.

Human growth hormone (HGH) is an unusual looking molecule, shaped somewhat like a snail sneaking into your garden late at night for a snack. It is composed of 191 amino acids strung together in a linear sequence with two loops formed by disulfide bridges (see Figure 7-3). Nothing about the appearance of this hormone would suggest to you either how important it is in vital growth processes, or its capacity to go awry and produce giants from ordinary folks.

It is nice to think about growth hormone as a single entity secreted from the anterior pituitary gland in response to various stimuli. In fact, however, a family of hormones similar in structure to the usual form of human growth hormone, and each of which may have different growth-promoting properties throughout the body, have recently been discovered in the pituitary gland. The role of these growth hormone variants remains to be uncovered.

Growth hormone secretion from the anterior pituitary gland is regulated by two—and as far as we know only two—hormones from the hypothalamus via the portal blood supply (shown in Figure 7-4). Somatostatin, a peptide composed of 14 amino acids, has an inhibitory effect on growth hormone release, while growth-hormone-releasing hormone (GHRH), composed of 40 amino acids, stimulates the synthesis and release of growth hormone from anterior pituitary cells. As we begin to explore the mechanisms by which somatostatin and GHRH are produced in the hypothalamus the story gets more complex. Stimuli from elsewhere in the brain are transmitted by the central nervous system to neurons in the hypothalamus that make somatostatin and GHRH, which then find their way into the portal circulation and regulate growth hormone release.

About one hour after the onset of sleep a major burst of growth hormone is released from the pituitary. Similar increases in growth hormone secretion also occur after exercise and when the blood glucose level is abruptly lowered by insulin. Throughout the day there are episodic peaks of growth hormone release, seemingly random, perhaps built in by the evolutionary tinkerer to add a touch of chaos to what would otherwise be a preposterously monotonous situation. Other pituitary hormones also exhibit episodic fluctuations, so there may be some utility lurking in the background. Certain substances such as arginine, glucagon, and L-dopa also cause growth hormone release, whereas high blood levels of glucose suppress growth hormone production. In all of these situations the stimulation or suppression of growth hormone release is presumably mediated through the hypothalamic neurons that make GHRH and somatostatin, so that growth hormone production is tightly regulated by the brain through the hypothalamus just as the other anterior pituitary hormones are.

Once released from the pituitary, how does growth hormone exert its effect? This still unanswered question has intrigued physicians and physiologists since the discovery of the hormone in the 1920s. When, in the 1930s, growth hormone became available from pituitary extracts, investigators began to study its effects on bone growth and metabolism in animals. It was soon recognized that the growth plates at the ends of bones grew very poorly in animals whose pituitary gland had been removed, but that growth could be restored to normal by injecting growth hormone. It was therefore assumed that growth hormone in some way acted directly on the bone to stimulate bone growth. However, several important experiments shattered this notion and replaced it with a speculative proposal that to this day is still being sorted out. It is referred to as the "somatomedin hypothesis."

This hypothesis arose out of the observation by Salmon and Daughaday that growth hormone by itself has no direct metabolic effects on bone cartilage. Rather, growth hormone leads to the appearance of growth factors (called *somatomedins*) in the serum, and these growth

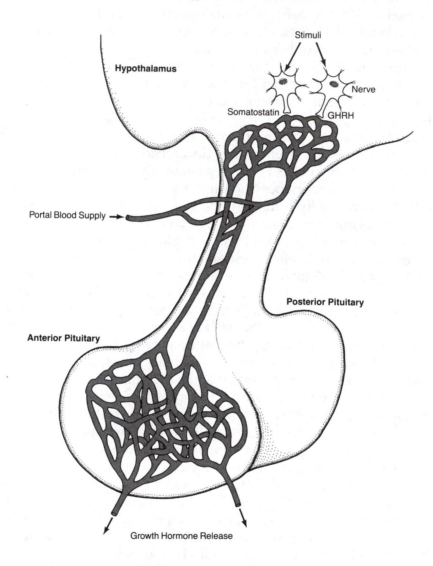

Figure 7-4. The release of growth hormone from the anterior pituitary is regulated by neurons in the hypothalamus that release GHRH and somatostatin into the portal blood supply.

factors are the substances that act on the cartilage to promote growth. The term "somatomedin" is now used to designate any substance that acts on cartilage and is regulated by growth hormone. In addition to their action on cartilage, the somatomedins also have other metabolic activities in the body such as insulin-like action on muscle and fat cells as well as growth stimulation of other cells.

The somatomedins originate primarily in the liver, where growth hormone stimulates their synthesis and release into the circulation. (They are peptide hormones with some resemblance to proinsulin, which probably accounts for their insulin-like actions on muscle and fat cells.) After release from the liver they circulate via the bloodstream. The somatomedin hypothesis suggests that these circulating substances are responsible for the major growth-promoting activity of growth hormone. The somatomedins have not yet been isolated in sufficient quantity to prove conclusively that they can promote the growth of animals or humans deficient in growth hormone itself. Recent experiments from Sweden indicate that growth hormone can also act directly on the bones of rats to promote growth, perhaps by stimulating local somatomedin production by bone cells. Continuing research should eventually establish the role of growth hormone and the somatomedins in the promotion of growth and perhaps uncover other, as yet unknown, important growth factors.

Future Therapeutics

The treatment of short children with growth hormone deficiency was revolutionized in the 1950s by the discovery that not just any growth hormone would do—the hormone had to come from human pituitaries and not from animals. Beck's demonstration of the striking metabolic effects of human growth hormone in a 13-year-old boy with a deficiency was followed by Raben's evidence that human growth hormone is effective in promoting the long-term growth of pituitary dwarfs. About one in every 5,000 children has growth hormone deficiency, a problem that can be corrected provided that the treatment is started early in life. It is imperative to recognize and treat this disorder at an early age. If treatment is started before five years of age, then full adult height can be anticipated, whereas by nine years of age only two-thirds of the height loss can be recovered. The supply of growth hormone has until now been extremely limited because it had to be isolated from the pituitary glands of human cadavers. Fortunately, this limited supply has matched up reasonably well with the infrequency of growth hormone deficiency as a cause of short stature, and most patients have been able to receive adequate treatment. The balance between the supply and demand for growth hormone has recently been jolted, however, from two different directions—the discovery that many more short children besides those suffering from growth hormone deficiency may benefit from this treatment, and the discovery that through the use of recombinant DNA technology human growth hormone can be synthesized in the laboratory by bacteria.

Rudman and his colleagues have recently studied in detail a set of children with what is designated as normal-variant short stature. By definition these children are all below the third percentile in height, have no apparent organic cause for their short stature, and show normal serum growth hormone levels by radioimmunoassay during provocative tests such as insulin-induced hypoglycemia. Normal-variant short stature is very common and occurs in about 40 percent of children who are below the third percentile in height. Rudman has shown that some of the children with normal-variant short stature have low serum somatomedin C levels and when treated with human growth hormone they exhibit accelerated growth—in some cases the results are quite similar to those achieved in children with growth hormone deficiency. This suggests that a much larger group of children with short stature may show increased growth with growth hormone therapy, perhaps as many as one in every 500 children. Whether or not these children *should* be treated with growth hormone is an entirely different question.

Fortunately a new source of human growth has become available: Recombinant DNA technology is used to insert the gene coding for growth hormone into the bacterium *Escherichia coli*. Investigators at Stanford and Genentech have shown that the human growth hormone analog synthesized by *E. coli* bacteria is equivalent in its metabolic activity to growth hormone isolated from human pituitaries in adults. Experiments are now under way to treat short children with the new human growth analog, and the results of these studies may well usher in a new era of therapy to promote growth in selected short children.

8

A TREATMENT FROM TORONTO

■

On December 2, 1921, a 13-year-old boy, Leonard Thompson, was admitted to the medical ward of Toronto General Hospital. Pale and undernourished, he weighed only 65 pounds. His blood pressure was low and he lacked energy. Blood and urine tests indicated that he had severe juvenile onset diabetes mellitus. After languishing in the hospital for over a month on a special diet, his clinical condition took a turn for the worse. There was little to suggest that he would survive this illness and become the focal point of a revolution that had been brewing for months in the Physiology Department at the University of Toronto.

There are occasional turning points in medicine when momentous laboratory discoveries have immediate clinical applications and this was just such a moment. Unknowingly, Leonard Thompson had picked the right time and the right place to suffer his affliction of severe diabetes mellitus. On January 11, 1922, he received an injection of an extract prepared from beef pancreas glands by Frederick Banting and Charles Best. They had been working diligently for eight months in the laboratory of J. J. MacLeod, trying to isolate insulin. The note in Thompson's hospital record was terse and to the point—"15 cc of MacLeod's serum. 7½ cc into each buttock." That's all, no fanfare, no indication that a medical milestone had been reached.

With this injection, Leonard Thompson's serum sugar level fell about 25 percent. Shortly afterward a more potent extract brought his serum sugar level down close to normal. These pancreas extracts contained the hormone insulin—the first available for human use. The patient was then placed on long-term insulin therapy and lived a relatively normal life for 14 more years before he died of pneumonia at the age of 27. Since the introduction of insulin into clinical practice in 1922, millions of diabetic patients have benefited from insulin therapy; they owe their lives to the pioneering research of Banting and Best and the many other investigators who have contributed to the isolation and purification of insulin. How did the discovery of insulin in the pancreas of animals unfold and why did it take so long to make this discovery?

The Discovery and Isolation of Insulin

Diabetes is an ancient disease; good clinical descriptions of the disorder are found in ancient Chinese, Hindu, and Greek writings that document the excessive urination, thirst, and weakness that are so characteristic of the affliction. About 100 A.D. the Greek physician Aretaeos coined the word *diabetes*, meaning "to pass through." Eventually the urine of diabetics was discovered to taste sweet, giving rise to the name *diabetes mellitus*. In the eighteenth century, Matthew Dobson in England ascertained that the urine and blood of diabetics actually do contain excessive amounts of sugar, and in 1815 Chevreul proved that the excessive sugar was glucose.

Still there were no hints about the cause of diabetes until observations began to trickle in on patients with injuries to the pancreas gland who developed diabetes. The pancreas gland is located behind the stomach and is connected to the first part of the small intestine (the duodenum) by a tube called the pancreatic duct. After the ingestion of food, the pancreas secretes a number of digestive enzymes into the small intestine through the pancreatic duct; this is called an *exocrine function*, an outward secretion through a duct, away from the bloodstream and internal body. This exocrine function of the pancreas, the secretion of digestive enzymes into the duodenum to help digest food, was already recognized in the seventeenth century. It was not until the late nineteenth century, however, that the *endocrine function* of the pancreas was recognized—the function that results in the internal secretion of insulin into the bloodstream to regulate the metabolism of nutrients throughout the body.

In 1869 a young German medical student named Paul Langerhans, in a thesis submitted for his M.D. degree, described some unusual clusters of cells scattered throughout the pancreas like galaxies in a pancreatic universe. He did not make much of this observation except to emphasize that these clusters of cells were entirely different in appearance from the surrounding pancreas cells. The idea that these islets of Langerhans (as they came to be called) performed an endocrine function did not arise until 24 years later, when Laguesse suggested that the cells in the islets secreted something that prevented diabetes mellitus—the first hypothesis of the existence of such a substance. The Laguesse hypothesis was made possible by the important experiments of Joseph von Mering and Oscar Minkowski, who had published their now classic observations on the development of diabetes mellitus in dogs after removal of their pancreas glands.

Originally von Mering and Minkowski were interested in the role of the pancreas in the digestion of fats, but when they meticulously removed the gland from a dog they were surprised to observe that the dog began to have a marked increase in urination. They tested the urine and were astonished to find a large amount of sugar present—an experimental model of diabetes mellitus had been inadvertently produced by removal of the pancreas, a gland that appeared in some way to be responsible for regulation of the blood sugar level. After others corroborated the discovery that removal of the pancreas in dogs and in other animals causes diabetes mellitus, the path was open for a search for the presumed regulator of the blood glucose level—a substance that eventually acquired the name "insulin." It was a tortuous road from the speculation by Laguesse in 1893 that the islets of Langerhans in the pancreas produced an internal secretion that regulates the blood sugar level to the isolation of insulin by Banting and Best in 1922.

Most of the numerous earlier attempts to prepare from animal pancreas glands extracts that could be injected into humans to lower the blood sugar level failed for one reason or another. In several noteworthy research efforts the investigators came up with results quite similar to the later results of Banting and Best. The first and certainly the most bizarre event in the quest to isolate insulin was initiated by the talented French physiologist, Eugene Gley, who in 1905 isolated pancreas extracts by a method nearly identical to that eventually used by Banting and Best. Gley injected the extracts into diabetic dogs, producing considerable improvement in their clinical condition. Here, 25 years before the breakthrough in Toronto, were virtually the same experiments that would be performed by Banting and Best. For reasons entirely mysterious, Gley refused to publish his results but rather sealed them in a packet which he deposited with the French Society of Biology in 1905, not to be opened until many years later. Gley had

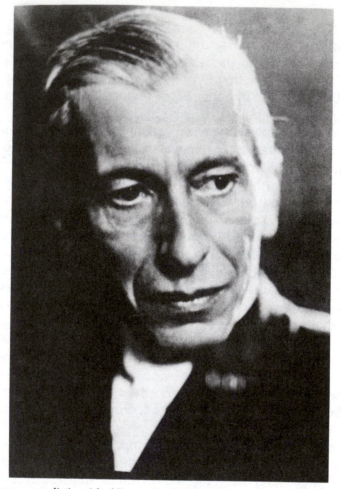

Nicolas Paulesco was a distinguished Rumanian physiologist who discovered insulin in pancreas extracts before the isolation of insulin by Banting and Best in 1921.

discovered insulin without knowing what he had done, simply too far ahead of his time to recognize the significance of his discovery.

The Rumanian Nicolas Paulesco was of another stripe. Paulesco was a distinguished professor of physiology at the school of medicine in Bucharest and over a period of 20 years had made important contributions to the field of pituitary physiology, including an ingenious neurosurgical technique to remove the pituitary gland from animals. In 1916 he discovered that pancreatic extracts injected into diabetic dogs produced a decrease in urination. After World War I he prepared extracts from dog and beef pancreas glands that lowered the sugar level in the blood and urine of diabetic dogs. He knew exactly what he was doing when he prepared pancreatic extracts that produced severe hypoglycemia (low blood sugar) in dogs. His extracts undoubtedly contained insulin, and Paulesco, recognizing the significance of his finding, published his results in August 1921—some six months before Banting and Best published their landmark paper on the isolation of insulin. After publishing these results in 1921, Paulesco set out to try to treat humans with pancreas extracts. But his work was surpassed by the efforts of the Toronto group, who purified insulin to an extent that made it possible to treat human patients.

Nevertheless, Paulesco's achievement was of great stature, sufficient, in the view of many, to warrant him a share of the Nobel Prize in 1923, which was awarded, however, only to Banting and MacLeod. The award set off a considerable furor not only in Rumania because of the exclusion of Paulesco, but also in Toronto because of the exclusion of Best, who performed the experiments on the isolation of insulin with Banting in MacLeod's laboratory. Those who take the Nobel Prize seriously will recognize this inequity as a recurring theme, inherent in the awarding of prizes for important discoveries—it is often difficult to determine just exactly who contributed what and when.

Frederick Banting and Charles Best were an unlikely pair to stumble upon the isolation of insulin; in contrast to Paulesco and MacLeod, neither had extensive experience in physiology research. They literally started from scratch without fully appreciating the difficulty of their task. Nor did they pay much attention to the previous 30 years of failure on the part of many investigators to isolate insulin from pancreas extracts.

The research project that culminated in the discovery of insulin began in obscurity. Banting was trained as an orthopedic surgeon, and in 1920 he tried to establish a general practice in London, Ontario. Because his practice was not lucrative, he worked part-time in the Department of Physiology at the University of Western Ontario. It was while preparing a lecture on diabetes that an idea occurred to him that was to become the turning point of his life—he surmised that previous investigators had been unable to isolate insulin from pancreas extracts because the enzymes in the exocrine portion of the pancreas gland destroyed the insulin molecule during the isolation procedure. He hit upon the idea of tying off the pancreatic duct near its entry into the duodenum, which he knew from previously published

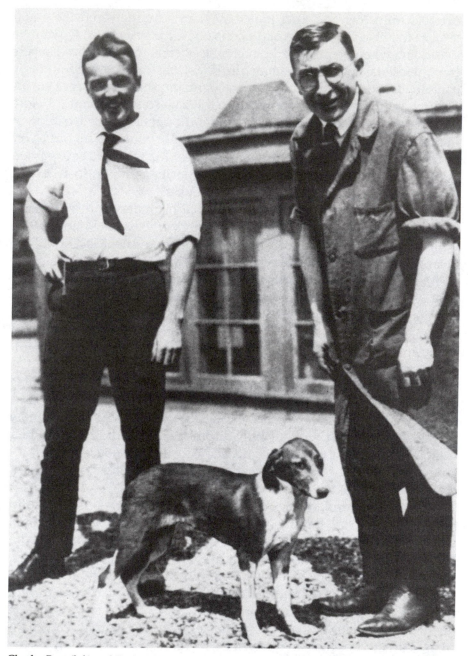

Charles Best (left) and Frederick Banting (right) are shown with one of their experimental dogs. During the summer and fall of 1921 Banting and Best isolated insulin from the pancreas of healthy dogs and used this insulin to keep diabetic dogs alive. The publication of their discovery and purification of insulin in February 1922 created a sensation in the medical community.

research would lead to degeneration of the exocrine pancreas, leaving behind the islets of Langerhans, where he presumed insulin was contained. Banting took his idea to J. J. MacLeod, who was the leading carbohydrate physiologist in Canada and a renowned expert in experimental diabetes. Although somewhat skeptical about the proposed experiments of the upstart young surgeon, MacLeod did offer him a laboratory in the medical building at Toronto University. MacLeod also assigned one of his physiology graduate students, Charles Best, to assist Banting on the project.

Best was raised in a small town in northern Maine, the son of a country doctor. At the age of twelve, he was assisting his father in administering anesthetics and generally showed an intense interest in medical subjects. His aunt, Anna Best, had diabetes mellitus and her death from diabetic coma had a considerable influence on his choice of a career in medical research. In May 1921 he embarked with Banting on their historic voyage to isolate insulin, an eight-month journey that brought them both international fame and opened up new vistas of life to millions of diabetics.

The research began in obscurity on a shoestring budget. They worked around the clock through the hot Toronto summer while MacLeod was away in Scotland. They lived in the laboratory, cooking over a Bunsen burner. Slowly they perfected their techniques for preparing pancreas extracts and making accurate blood glucose measurements in the few experimental dogs available. Banting sold his car to help pay for supplies and food. Progress was slow, but by the end of July they had demonstrated that the extracts contained a substance that *did* lower the blood glucose level of diabetic dogs. When MacLeod returned from Scotland in September, he was astounded to find the two young investigators on the verge of a major discovery. He swung the full weight of his laboratory resources behind the project, and the experiments were repeated over and over until more than 75 successful experiments using a variety of techniques had demonstrated the capability of the pancreas extracts to lower blood sugar. Their findings were first presented at the University of Toronto in November and published for the world at large in February 1922.

MacLeod then secured the assistance of the biochemist J. B. Collip to help prepare purified insulin extracts for use in humans. Insulin therapy for the first human patient was begun in January 1922, and a new era in the treatment of diabetes was opened. Ultimately new and purified preparations of insulin were discovered and are now routinely

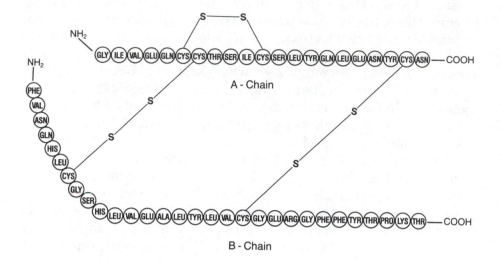

Human Insulin

Figure 8-1. Insulin is initially synthesized as proinsulin in beta cells located in the islets of Langerhans throughout the pancreas. Before being packaged into secretory granules, the proinsulin is converted to insulin which is composed of two chains of amino acids bound together by disulfide (-S-S-) bridges.

available for the treatment of diabetic patients. Large-scale production of purified insulin from pigs and cattle for the lifesaving treatment of diabetic patients throughout the world quickly followed. The chemical structure of insulin (see Figure 8-1) was completed in 1953. Recently, as recombinant DNA techniques have been developed to synthesize pure human insulin in bacteria, a new source of insulin has become available for clinical use.

The Role of Insulin

Insulin is the premiere storage hormone, designed to store nutrients for lean times, when no food is available—an ideal hormone for any species that fought its way through an evolutionary struggle where access to food was probably intermittent at best. Under these conditions it is of considerable value to be able to store away glucose as glycogen, amino acids as protein, and fatty acids as triglycerides. Investigators studying how insulin works, what regulates its secretion, and where it acts on the body turned their attention to the role of insulin in the metabolism of carbohydrate, protein, and fat. The knowledge they gained led to an increased understanding of the part insulin plays in the normal body economy.

Insulin is a small peptide hormone released into the circulation from the pancreas following the intake of food. The glucose and amino acids in the food stimulate synthesis and release of insulin from the islets of Langerhans by mechanisms still unidentified. The islets have a complexity all their own, as shown in Figure 8-2. A core of insulin-producing beta cells is surrounded by a rim of glucagon-producing alpha cells and a scattered set of delta cells that make somatostatin (the same hormone that is made in the hypothalamus to inhibit growth hormone secretion from the pituitary). Glucagon, as we shall see in more detail, has metabolic effects opposed to the metabolic effects of insulin, while somatostatin produced in the islets probably has direct inhibitor effects on both the alpha and beta cells.

When the blood glucose level increases—as it does following a meal containing carbohydrate—the beta cells respond by producing insulin, which tends to restore the glucose level toward normal, while glucagon production by alpha cells is suppressed. Conversely, during a fasting state, the insulin output is diminished and glucagon release is enhanced. In juvenile onset diabetes mellitus (now called type I diabetes mellitus) the beta cells are defective and do not produce an adequate amount of insulin; the blood glucose level therefore becomes elevated. Thus, the integrity of the islets of Langerhans has great importance for the preservation of normal metabolism.

Released into the bloodstream from the pancreas, insulin circulates to its important target sites—the liver, muscle, and fat tissues. These are the three primary places of action for insulin, which, like other peptide hormones, binds to receptors on the surface of cells and thereby initiates a cascade of biochemical events designed to store nutrients for later use. We have seen that insulin (or a molecule very much like it) appeared low down on the evolutionary ladder in bacteria and fungi, performing some mysterious unknown function. The higher organisms have cleverly utilized this molecule as a messenger, a signal from the islets of Langerhans to the liver, fat, and muscle tissues that it is time to store some nutrients away, to gear up for a time when food is not available. So we are stuck, for better or for worse, with the scheme depicted in Figure 8-3, in which insulin regulates intricate biochemical processes at the three target sites in a way that coordinates the overall storage of nutrients. Let us examine each

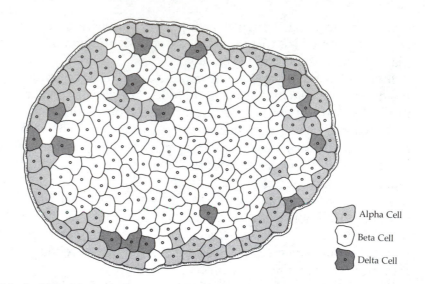

Alpha Cell

Beta Cell

Delta Cell

Figure 8-2. An islet of Langerhans in the pancreas is composed of three types of cells. The majority are beta cells which make insulin. They are surrounded by alpha cells which make glucagon and delta cells which make the hypothalamic hormone somatostatin.

of these target sites in somewhat more detail, looking into the interior of cells, reaching around in the nooks and crannies of the second messengers, enzyme cascades, and mitochondrial transfers to discern how it is that a molecule like insulin can have such a vast impact on the body's metabolic needs.

Let us begin at the liver, the first site of action for insulin after it leaves the pancreas. We start at the cell-surface receptors for insulin, those regions of the liver cell plasma membrane that show strong affinity for insulin. There is plenty of evidence that high-affinity insulin receptors exist on the surface of liver cells, and it is very likely that the action of insulin is initiated at the surface of the cell by interaction between insulin and its receptor. Beyond this interaction, however, little is known about the mechanism of insulin action; we do know that it is certainly not mediated by cyclic AMP like most other peptide hormones. The second messenger for insulin action (inside of cells) has remained uniquely difficult to identify; various candidates have come and gone, such as cyclic nucleotides, calcium ion, and other intracellular entities. Most recently a low-molecular-weight peptide has been identified as a possible second messenger for insulin action, but considerably more work needs to be done to expand this finding. In the meantime we are left with the concept that insulin most likely

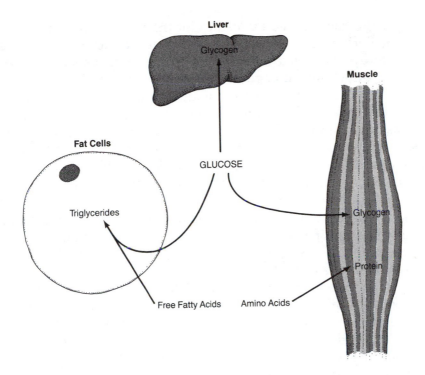

Figure 8-3. Insulin regulates the storage of fuel at three different sites in the body. Glucose is stored as glycogen, fatty acids as triglycerides, and amino acids as protein.

works like other peptide hormones—that is, it binds to the cell-surface receptor, which leads to the synthesis of a second messenger inside the cell and thereby initiates a whole cascade of chemical reactions to effect the precise action intended. In the case of the liver, the action intended is the storage of glucose into glycogen and of fatty acids into triglycerides, as well as the utilization of glucose to synthesize new fatty acids.

Glucose is an essential fuel for the functioning of the brain; the liver and muscles produce glucose for the brain when none is available as food. The synthesis of glycogen from glucose and the reverse reaction, the breakdown of glycogen to yield glucose, are each controlled by separate enzymes. During the first 12 hours of a fast and during muscular exercise, the breakdown of glycogen provides the major source of glucose. There is method in the madness: These chemical reactions are coordinated by insulin for the purpose of storing away nutrients such as glycogen and fat, to be used later when the food supply abruptly drops to zero and the next meal is nowhere in sight.

Insulin directs the storage of triglycerides inside of individual fat cells in the adipose tissue. Once again, insulin begins its regulation of the interior of the fat by first binding to a high-affinity receptor on the plasma membrane. This event sparks the production of a second messenger, undoubtedly the same mysterious elusive second messenger that controls the nutrient storage reactions inside of the liver and muscle cells. Inside of the fat cell the still unidentified second messenger initiates the conversion of free fatty acids into triglycerides by regulating a coordinated set of chemical reactions. It is clear that insulin plays a profound role in the storage of triglycerides; everything is coordinated for the purpose of storing up fats to be utilized as a fuel when there is a shortage of food.

Finally, in muscle cells insulin stimulates the uptake of glucose and the storage of glucose as glycogen. Insulin also stimulates the synthesis of protein and inhibits the breakdown of protein into its component amino acids. Here again, the whole program is orchestrated by an intracellular second messenger arising directly from the binding of insulin to receptors located on the muscle cell surface.

Insulin is a storage hormone that promotes the accumulation of glycogen, triglycerides, and protein in liver, fat, and muscle cells at a time when food is plentiful. Eating results indirectly in the production of insulin by beta cells located in the islets of Langerhans in the pancreas. During a prolonged fast the serum insulin falls to low levels, with a consequent release of glucose from glycogen, fatty acids and glycerol from triglycerides, and amino acids from protein—all to be used as metabolic fuels to keep the body running until food once again becomes available. Diabetes mellitus results when the beta cells are defective or when insulin does not work properly at its target sites.

The Maltese Faster

On April 10, 1912, the famous Mr. L marched into the metabolic laboratory of the Carnegie Institute to meet Dr. Francis Benedict and begin a 31-day total fast. That fast would lead to a classic publication on the detailed metabolic consequences of a prolonged period of food deprivation. Mr. L was a 40-year-old lawyer, who, in his native country of Malta, had founded the Society of Psychical Studies and Research— devoted to fasting as a treatment for a variety of afflictions—and had

TABLE 8-1

Body Fuel Origin	Body Fuels of the Average Sized Human		
	Weight (kg)	Calories	Percent Fuel
Fat	15.0	141,000	85.0
Protein	6.0	24,000	14.0
Glycogen	0.225	900	0.5

himself considerable experiences of fasting. The idea that a lawyer would donate his body to medical science might rattle the biases of anyone looking at the present day interactions of the medical and legal professions, but this was a different era and Mr. L a different kind of lawyer.

He was not the first person to hit upon the notion that fasting had therapeutic value. Fasting has been extolled throughout history by many different religious sects. In ancient Greece fasting was popular as a means of arousing visions and making contact with supernatural forces. In the nineteenth century numerous books and medical publications reported the effects of prolonged fasting. But the detailed metabolic and physical studies Benedict performed during the 31-day fast of Mr. L were the first to lay a firm scientific foundation for understanding the metabolic consequences of prolonged food deprivation. Mr. L ate no food for 31 days; during this period Benedict and a bevy of lab assistants measured all organic and inorganic waste products for which good tests were available. They frequently monitored Mr. L's oxygen consumption and carbon dioxide production and did meticulous metabolic balance studies, employing a large clumsy apparatus (total body calorimeter) specially designed for the purpose.

Benedict showed that during the first several days of the fast all of Mr. L's carbohydrate stores were consumed, and during the rest of the fast Mr. L lived off his fat and protein stores, with the fat providing about 85 percent of his daily caloric requirement and protein about 15 percent. Mr. L's weight dropped from 132 pounds to 104 pounds, and his daily caloric requirement shifted from an initial level of 1,600 calories per day to about 1,300 calories per day at the end of the fast. His protein was increasingly conserved as he progressed through the fast, as evidenced by a fall in the daily excretion of nitrogen in his urine. Thus, during a prolonged fast, the glycogen stores are used up immediately, the protein losses are reduced to a minimum, and the fat stores are utilized as the primary source of fuel. A glance at Table

TABLE 8-2

| Fasting Time (days) | Serum Glucose and Hormone Levels During Prolonged Fasting | | | |
	Glucose (ng/dl)[a]	Insulin (uU/ml)[b]	Glucagon (pg/ml)[c]	Growth Hormone (ng/ml)[d]
0	96	13.5	139	0.7
5	63	2.9	222	2.9
12	74	5.3	162	4.1
19	71	2.6	249	8.0
26	77	1.5	328	9.9
33	76	1.3	728	3.1

[a] milligrams per deciliter [b] microunits per milliliter [c] picograms per milliliter [d] nanograms per milliliter

8-1 demonstrates why the body has chosen this strategy—the vast majority of the fuel is stored in the fat tissue. Furthermore, most of the body protein is utilized for essential structural, mechanical, and enzymatic functions in muscle and other tissues; it is clearly economical to conserve the protein for these functions rather than expending the protein as a fuel.

The mobilization of fuel during fasting is regulated by hormones, and insulin is central to this scheme. As we have seen, the fundamental role of insulin in regulating the body's metabolism is to enhance the storage of nutrients in the form of glycogen, triglyceride, and protein. The marked fall in the serum insulin level caused by a prolonged fast results in a decreased storage of nutrients. Simultaneously there occurs an increase in counterregulatory hormones that promote glucose synthesis in the liver, such as glucagon from the pancreatic alpha cells in the islets of Langerhans, growth hormone and ACTH from the pituitary, and cortisol and epinephrine from the adrenal glands. These counterregulatory hormones oppose the action of insulin and stimulate the breakdown of the stored nutrients into circulating fuels that can be used by the brain, muscles, and other tissues for their caloric and metabolic requirements. These complex events are illustrated in Table 8-2 and Figure 8-3, which show that insulin and the counterregulatory hormones orchestrate the interaction among the liver, adipose, and muscle tissues to provide the body with essential fuels, glucose, and ketones during a prolonged fast.

The Problem of Hypoglycemia

When one is inclined to take a short-sighted view of the world from the vantage point of an endocrinologist, it appears as though we are witnessing an epidemic of hypoglycemia, a condition that results when the glucose concentration in the blood falls to a very low level. Patients develop symptoms of brain dysfunction—personality changes, seizures, assorted behaviors that border on the bizarre—and other unusual symptoms. It is perhaps a fundamental condition of modern existential life that many people need something tangible to blame for their unusual symptoms and behaviors, some legitimate explanation to explain the unexplainable. There is nothing like hypoglycemia to explain away a myriad of troubling feelings and behaviors. Fads in diagnosis, like fads in nutrition, come and go, fading slowly as the incoming children reject the myths, dogmas, and life styles of the outgoing parents. The present epidemic of hypoglycemia has resulted from a curious sloppiness in diagnosis by the medical profession. Time grinds down the aberrations from truth, and this will certainly be the fate of our present hypoglycemic era.

True cases of hypoglycemia do exist, but they are exceedingly rare. These cases often arise from tumors, either islet cell tumors in the pancreas that make excess insulin or tumors elsewhere in the body that produce substances that act like insulin. All of the types of tumors associated with hypoglycemia are rare. Hypoglycemia can result when glucose production by the liver is defective, either from intrinsic abnormalities in the liver or because counterregulatory hormones like cortisol and growth hormone are absent. Some drugs other than insulin can cause hypoglycemia. All in all, however, the causes of true hypoglycemia are limited in scope and are so infrequent that, in the everyday world of illness, hypoglycemia is rarely encountered except in diabetic patients who are on insulin therapy.

Diabetes Mellitus

The period immediately following the isolation of insulin by Banting and Best was a time of considerable enthusiasm in the treatment of diabetes mellitus. New methods to purify insulin were discovered and new types of insulin preparations were introduced into practice. Eliot Joslin, who established a famous clinic in Boston to treat diabetics, suggested, along with others, that tight regulation of blood glucose levels in diabetics might prevent some of the long-term complications of diabetes mellitus such as blindness and kidney failure. An immediate increase in the life expectancy of patients with the severe form of diabetes mellitus was possible because of the improvement in the treatment of *diabetic ketoacidosis*, a condition that, because of the lack of insulin, can result in coma and death.

It is not clear even today whether insulin therapy can prevent long-term complications; this is one of the key problems occupying the attention of investigators around the world. Do the long-term complications of diabetes mellitus—retina damage, kidney failure, accelerated atherosclerosis with damage to the heart, and nerve damage—all result from elevation of the blood glucose level? Before considering the answer to this question, we will briefly review the etiology of diabetes mellitus and the nature of the long-term complications associated with the disorder.

The term "diabetes mellitus" actually applies to a number of different disorders whose common characteristic is an elevated blood glucose level. The diagnosis is not that difficult to make: You stay out of the refrigerator after dinner one evening and hold yourself in a fasting state until the following morning, when you have a blood specimen drawn. If your plasma glucose level is 140 mg/dl or greater, then you've got diabetes mellitus.

There are two major types of diabetes mellitus. The first type is called insulin-dependent diabetes mellitus (IDDM) or simply type I diabetes mellitus; this type usually has its onset in childhood or in young adults. Type I is characterized by low serum insulin levels and absolutely requires insulin therapy. Without insulin therapy the type I diabetic will decompensate into hyperglycemia (high blood glucose level) and ketoacidosis, in which the ketones normally reproduced at a low level during starvation to provide fuel for brain and muscle cells now accumulate excessively in the bloodstream and become a threat to the patient's life. The synthesis of ketones from fatty acids in the liver is normally regulated by insulin and glucagon; when the serum insulin level is very low and the glucagon level high, as in type I diabetes mellitus, then ketone production by the liver is at a maximum. Without insulin, the type I diabetic will not survive long, and it is these diabetics who have benefited the most from the discovery and purification of insulin.

The second major type of diabetes mellitus is called non-insulin-dependent diabetes mellitus (NIDDM) or just type II diabetes mellitus. Whereas type I diabetes seems to result from the damage to beta cells by immune reactions or virus infections, with a consequent low serum insulin level, the cause of type II diabetes is more complex. Type II usually occurs in persons over the age of 40 and is characterized by a resistance to insulin at the target tissues in combination with defective function of beta cells in the pancreas. Type II diabetics do not develop ketoacidosis in the absence of insulin therapy but have variable degrees of elevated blood glucose levels. The condition is often aggravated by obesity and may be markedly improved by dieting down to ideal body weight. Thus, many type II diabetic patients require neither insulin therapy nor the oral antidiabetic pills in order to adequately control the disorder.

Diabetes mellitus will also result from any disease, such as pancreatitis or hemochromatosis, which severely damages the pancreas. And, of course, if the pancreas is surgically removed for any reason, diabetes mellitus will occur. Some drugs can cause diabetes mellitus by increasing resistance to insulin or by inhibiting the release of insulin from the pancreas. In short, there are many different ways to develop diabetes mellitus.

If the treatment of diabetes mellitus were only a matter of regulating the blood glucose level within a range that prevented hyperglycemic coma at one extreme and hypoglycemic insulin reactions at the other extreme, then the disease would pose few major clinical problems and the life expectancy of most diabetic patients would probably be similar to that of the general population. Unfortunately, the development of disease in the blood vessels and nerves threatens the well-being of diabetics. Small blood vessels in the eyes, kidneys, and at other sites in the body become progressively narrowed as the duration of the illness increases; after many years these changes can lead to decreased vision, diminished kidney function, and poor circulation in the extremities. An acceleration of atherosclerosis in diabetes narrows large blood vessels in the body (due to the deposition of atherosclerotic plaques) and these changes can result in poor circulation to the heart, brain, and legs as well as to other organ systems. Finally, diabetes is associated with damage to the autonomic, peripheral, and sensory nerves. All of these complications of the blood vessels and nerves often make the management of the diabetic patient an exceedingly complex ordeal, requiring the utmost attention to detail by the patient and by the physician.

The central working hypothesis of most diabetes specialists at the present time is that blood vessel and nerve abnormalities seen in association with diabetes mellitus result directly from the elevated blood glucose levels. If the glucose level could be tightly controlled, as it is in nondiabetic persons who have normally functioning pancreatic beta cells, then the blood vessels and nerves would not be damaged. This hypothesis is not just a whim of well-meaning physicians and scientists working on the problem of diabetes. There are good studies in animals to strongly support the hypothesis. For example, diabetic rats develop kidney disease that completely disappears when the rats are rendered non-diabetic by pancreas transplants. The kidney disease also disappears when the diabetic kidney is transplanted into a normal rat. Similarly, nerve conduction in diabetic rats can be markedly improved by tightly controlling the rats' blood glucose levels. Studies on humans are to date contradictory: Some show improvement in kidney and eye disease with tight glucose control, but several recent studies have shown short-term worsening of eye disease in patients whose blood glucose levels are tightly controlled.

Although many recent advances in the technology of glucose control have been made, none of the methodologies—including elaborate home glucose-monitoring techniques and expensive portable insulin infusion pumps—are able to duplicate the exquisitely tight control of a normal pancreas gland. When we eventually have available devices that can simulate the glucose control of a normal pancreas, then perhaps we will witness the next major revolution in the management of diabetic patients—namely the simultaneous return to normal of elevated blood glucose levels and the cessation of the dreaded long-term complications of diabetes. The therapy of diabetes, which began with the discovery and purification of insulin, will then have come full circle, with the virtual elimination of diabetes as we presently know it—a disorder that presently affects over 10 million people in the United States. And, beyond this successful treatment, progress in understanding the cause of the various types of diabetes could eventually lead to the prevention of its onset. Progress of this kind in therapy and prevention will arise only through a persistent, tenacious, well-funded research effort.

9

BONES AND STONES

∎

Upon graduation at the top of his class from the Massachusetts Nautical School in 1916, Captain Charles Martell became a master mariner in the United States Merchant Marine. At the time of the Armistice in November 1918, he stood 6 feet 1 inch tall and was about to begin his own heroic struggle with a new and unusual metabolic bone disease that would require numerous hospitalizations, seven operations, and a plethora of ineffectual remedies lasting over a period of 14 years. His illness began, as chronic diseases often do, in a very subtle fashion, and resulted in slowly increasing disability. Pain in his back and legs was the initial symptom, and then he began to shrink—7 inches between 1918 and 1926.

In addition to losing height, he became pigeon-breasted and began to pass a white gravel in his urine. A series of unexpected bone fractures in the knees and arms followed, along with a series of incorrect diagnoses. The captain was literally falling apart at the seams; some unusual process was chipping away at the infrastructure—his bones were disappearing along with his height and his skeletal integrity. He was subjected to various inept treaments, including radiated milk, epinephrine, vegetable diets, and heliotherapy, all to no avail.

Finally, Martell ended up at Bellevue Hospital in New York City, where he had the good fortune to encounter Dr. Eugene DuBois, who took an exceptional interest in his case. DuBois discovered for the first time that Captain Martell had a very high level of calcium in his blood; a calcium-balance study further demonstrated that the captain was excreting far more calcium than he was consuming in his diet. From these metabolic abnormalities and from his knowledge of some obser-

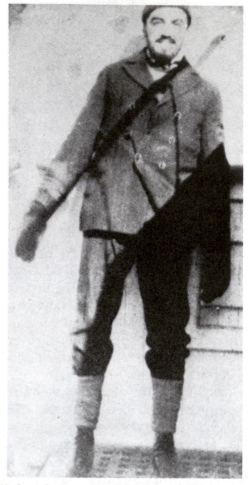

Captain Martell in 1918 about the time of his first symptoms of hyperparathyroidism.

vations on normal subjects who had been injected with parathyroid hormone extracts at Massachusetts General Hospital, DuBois concluded that the captain was suffering from the overproduction of parathyroid hormone, a condition he designated as *hyperparathyroidism*—the first such diagnosis in the United States.

About the same time as DuBois's discovery, a Viennese surgeon named Felix Mandl noted a patient with similar severe wasting of the bones. Mandl operated on his patient and discovered a benign tumor of one of the parathyroid glands. When he removed the tumor, the patient made a remarkable recovery. Captain Martell underwent six neck operations, but no parathyroid tumor was uncovered. He persisted, however, in subjecting himself to various research protocols. He studied everything he could get his hands on about hyperparathyroidism and the anatomy of the parathyroid glands. Finally, the captain concluded from his own anatomical studies that he had a parathyroid tumor in an aberrant location. Normally there are four parathyroid glands in humans, located in the neck just behind the thyroid gland, but occasionally the system goes awry and one of the parathyroid glands ends up in the chest. The captain urged the surgeons to open up his chest to search for the evasive parathyroid tumor; and so in November 1932, some 14 years after the onset of his first symptoms of bone pain, he underwent chest exploration that revealed a large parathyroid tumor. When this was removed, his serum calcium level fell rapidly and his bones began to improve. Unfortunately, he died about six weeks after removal of the tumor from the complications of a kidney stone.

Captain Martell had undergone a heroic struggle to find a cure for his affliction, and in the process of his courageous efforts the physiology of parathyroid hormone excess was elucidated by medical researchers in New York and at the Massachusetts General Hospital in Boston. From this one patient practically all the features of hyperparathyroidism were revealed, including the possibility of aberrant locations of parathyroid tumors. When parathyroid hormone is produced in excess by a parathyroid tumor, the bones begin to waste away, resulting in bone pain, fractures, and loss of height due to vertebral body collapse. The calcium is leached out of the bones by parathyroid hormone and is excreted in the urine, which leads to the formation of kidney stones. How was the connection between the parathyroid glands and calcium metabolism established, and how does the parathyroid work to maintain calcium balance?

The Parathyroids and Calcium Regulation

The parathyroid glands remained hidden from view for thousands of years. Not until the middle of the nineteenth century did awareness of their existence slowly emerge, by serendipity, from a morass of anatomical studies. The first hints came from Richard Owen in England, who was doing some anatomical studies of an Indian rhinoceros. If one were ever going to discover the existence of some very small glands in an obscure location, the rhino is not a bad place to start and, indeed, Owen noticed a small yellowish gland attached to the thyroid on the rhino's neck. This observation was more or less ignored until Yvar Sandstroem performed detailed neck dissections in 50 human cadavers and was able to demonstrate in most dissections four glands attached to the thyroid, two on each side of the neck. He called these "parathyroid glands" because of their location next to the thyroid gland, although, as it turns out, the parathyroid glands have no functional relationship to the thyroid gland. The parathyroids secrete *parathyroid hormone* (PTH), which regulates the blood calcium level within narrow limits; the thyroid secretes thyroxine, which controls the rate of metabolism of many different cells throughout the body. At the time of their discovery by Sandstroem in 1880, the connection between the parathyroid glands and calcium metabolism was unknown.

Sandstroem's discovery was basically ignored by the scientific community and had to be exhumed by the French physiologist Gley, who, along with other investigators in the late nineteenth and early twentieth centuries, noted that when their parathyroids were completely removed, animals developed *tetany*, a condition in which many different muscle groups go into spasm. It was natural to conclude that the parathyroid glands elaborated something that prevented muscles from twitching; but the idea that they elaborated a hormone that prevented the blood calcium from falling to dangerously low levels had to await a further series of important experiments by researchers in Europe and the United States.

The observation by Jacques Loeb at the Rockefeller Institute in New York that calcium prevented frog muscles from twitching was followed by a series of experiments in Vienna by Jacob Erdheim, who demonstrated that when the parathyroid glands were removed from rats, calcium was not deposited in growing teeth; they became fragile and broke easily. Up to this point, then, there seemed to be an intimate relationship among the parathyroid glands, calcium metabolism, and the phenomenon of tetany. To pull this labyrinth of twitching muscles and rotting teeth together, further key experiments were necessary, and these were supplied by two young investigators at Johns Hopkins University at Baltimore, MacCallum and Voegtlin. They removed the parathyroid glands from dogs; this, as others had shown, led to tetany. But they went on to show that the blood of these dogs contained a low level of calcium and that when calcium was injected into the blood of dogs, the tetany disappeared. Here was proof that the parathyroids in some way maintained the blood calcium concentration at a normal level, that removal of the parathyroids resulted in a low calcium level and tetany, and that the tetany could be cured by injecting calcium into the dogs.

Other investigators confirmed these results in animals and expanded the observations to humans who developed symptoms of tetany when they lost the function of their parathyroid glands. Tetany could be cured either by calcium-rich diets or by transplants of parathyroid grafts. As more accurate methods for measuring blood and urine calcium levels were developed, the physiology of calcium regulation could be studied in a more quantitative way. The normal range for the serum calcium level in humans was discovered to be about 9 to 11 milligrams per 100 milliliters. In patients who had lost their parathyroid glands from thyroid surgery or other causes, the level dropped to about 5.5 milligrams per 100 milliliters, with the simultaneous development of spasms and other signs of tetany.

It was now apparent that the parathyroid glands secrete a hormone that regulates the serum calcium level within a narrow normal range, and a search for this hormone in parathyroid extracts began. Typically, the discovery of parathyroid hormone was simultaneously achieved by two different investigators, Adolph Hanson and J. B. Collip, working independently. They were both able to extract parathyroid hormone from the parathyroid glands of cattle by boiling the glands in a dilute solution of hydrochloric acid. Injection of this extract into dogs whose parathyroid glands had been removed caused a marked increase of the serum calcium level and prevented the dogs from developing tetany. Collip also demonstrated that when dogs were given an excess of parathyroid hormone extract they developed very high serum levels of calcium. These experiments left no doubt about the existence of parathyroid hormone, although it took another 50 years of research to uncover its exact chemical structure.

While the physiology of calcium regulation by parathyroid hormone was being elucidated in the United States, a series of intriguing observations related to the parathyroid glands was accumulating in Europe. An unusual bone disease, *osteitis fibrosa cystica*, characterized by fibrous deposits, cysts, and nests of giant cells inside of bones, was first described near the end of the nineteenth century. The cause of this disorder was unknown, but soon a number of patients with osteitis fibrosa cystica were discovered at autopsy to have a tumor of one of the parathyroid glands. Ultimately it was proposed that the parathyroid tumor somehow caused the bone disease. It was in 1925 that the Viennese surgeon Mandl decided to do a neck operation on a patient named Albert (the family name has never been divulged), who was suffering from osteitis fibrosa.

Albert's situation was remarkably similar to that of Captain Martell—his illness started with pain in the legs and hips and gradually became worse. He lost his job as a streetcar conductor and settled in for a long downhill decline. Like Captain Martell, he was subjected to a host of ineffectual treatments, including cod liver oil and mud baths. X-rays showed that his bones were becoming thin and contained cysts. After four years of this illness, he was unable to walk or stand because of severe bone pain, and he developed a white sediment in his urine. Injections of parathyroid extract made matters worse. In an act of desperation, Mandl finally took Albert to neck surgery, where a large parathyroid tumor was discovered and removed. Albert improved rapidly, with considerable healing of his bones; he was able to return to a functional life as a result of this landmark operation.

As we noted, a similar operation had been tried on Captain Martell, but no parathyroid tumor was found until years later, when it was discovered in his upper chest. Nevertheless, the cases of Martell and Albert, along with several others in the late 1920s, led to the identification and cure of hyperparathyroidism, as well as to a deeper understanding of the intimate relationship between parathyroid hormone, bone metabolism, and calcium regulation. The details of just how and where parathyroid hormone acts to maintain the serum calcium at exactly the right level would begin to unfold over the subsequent decades and is today revealing ever deepening levels of complexity.

Regulation of Calcium Metabolism

Calcium is essential for the existence of all higher organisms. It is bonded with phosphate as an insoluble mineral to form bone, the structural framework for many different animals. Calcium also exists as an ion in the blood, in various other body fluids, and inside of cells, where it regulates important metabolic events. These two pools of calcium, the insoluble pool in bones and the calcium ion pool in body fluids, are not independent but rather are in delicate equilibrium with each other. Under circumstances where the serum calcium ion concentration would tend to fall to low levels—when, for example, too little calcium is present in the diet—calcium is leached from bones to keep the serum calcium level normal, a process that is mediated by parathyroid hormone and vitamin D. The bones are sacrificed to preserve the calcium ion concentration in body fluids, and this explains why the bones become thin (*osteoporosis*) in people who do not consume an adequate amount of calcium in their diet.

Bone is a complex dynamic tissue, constantly remodeling as new bone is laid down in layered strips and old bone is resorbed. These tasks are accomplished largely by two types of bone cells, the *osteoblasts*, which synthesize new bone matrix, and the *osteoclasts*, which resorb bone. The activities of bone synthesis by osteoblasts and bone resorption by osteoclasts are tightly linked (by unknown mechanisms), so that the dynamic remodeling of bone is kept in balance. During the growth period of early life, there is a net positive balance in calcium as bones grow to attain full maturation, while during the senescent phase of life—after the age of 30—there is a slight negative calcium balance, leading to the loss of bone from the body. About 99 percent of the body's calcium is stored in skeletal bone, while the remaining 1 percent is found as calcium ions in fluids and cells elsewhere in the body. Parathyroid hormone is one of the major regulators of the flow of calcium into and out of bone. When the hormone is absent, bone resorption is impaired and the serum calcium concentration falls to a dangerously low level; when the hormone is present in excess the serum calcium level may become dangerously elevated.

Calcium ions are extremely important in the functioning of many cells and processes throughout the body, so that any disturbances of normal calcium ion concentrations can have a profound impact. These ions are necessary for normal nerve signal transmission and muscle cell contractions. They are essential for blood clotting and for the secretion of hormones from many different cells. Recently it has become apparent that calcium may also be involved in the functioning of cell membranes and the action of peptide hormones at their target sites. Given this multitude of important functions, it is no wonder that the serum concentration of calcium is so tightly regulated within narrow limits. Low levels of serum calcium are associated with muscle spasms, cramps, seizures, and anxiety, whereas elevated levels lead to mental lethargy, depression, nausea, constipation, and, ultimately, calcification of the kidneys.

The serum calcium level is regulated by the concerted action of parathyroid hormone (PTH) and vitamin D (see Figure 9-1). The absorption of dietary calcium is mediated by vitamin D, an important chemical that enhances the synthesis of a calcium-binding protein located in cells lining the small intestine. This protein transports cal-

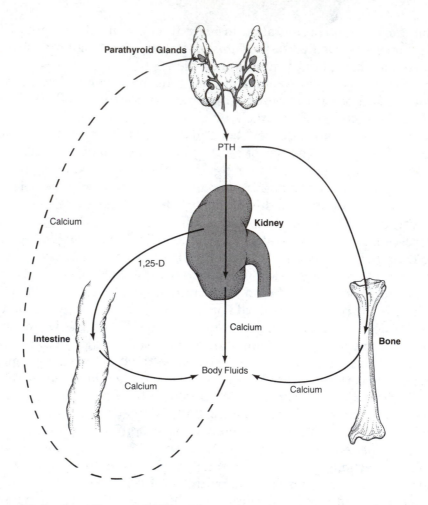

Figure 9-1. Parathyroid hormone (PTH) and the vitamin D metabolite 1,25(OH)$_2$D$_3$ regulate the flow of calcium from bone, kidneys, and intestine into the circulation.

cium from the intestine to the circulation. A derivative of vitamin D (called 1,25-dihydroxyvitamin D) is actually responsible for stimulating synthesis of the binding protein and, interestingly, PTH promotes synthesis of this derivative. Thus a deficiency in either PTH or vitamin D leads to poor absorption of calcium from the gut. A second point of regulation of calcium metabolism occurs in the kidneys, where small amounts of calcium are excreted into the urine each day. PTH stimulates cells in the kidney tubules to resorb calcium back into the circulation. When PTH is absent, a considerable quantity of calcium can be lost in the urine until the serum calcium concentration falls to a low level. Finally, PTH acts on bone in concert with vitamin D to release calcium into the bloodstream; this serves as a buffer to prevent a fall in calcium level at times when calcium is not being consumed in the diet.

Vitamin D

The discovery that vitamin D is essential for the normal calcification of bones in growing children and in adults took nearly 300 years to unfold. In the 1600s, Daniel Whistler and Francis Glisson independently of each other described a unique disease in English children called *rickets*. The illness in its severest form was devastating, resulting in dwarfed children with prominent frontal bones of the head and crooked leg bones. Conspicuous knobs of bone were present in the ribs and wrists, and the children showed a considerable degree of lassitude associated with muscle weakness and laxity of the joints. At the time of these early initial observations there were no hints as to the cause of the affliction.

There was little progress in understanding rickets until the nineteenth century, when a series of observations on the histology of rachitic bone revealed an abnormal proliferation of uncalcified bone. It was further recognized that the adult version of the illness, called *osteomalacia*, also resulted from poor calcification of bone matrix, although in adults the bone became fragile and painful but did not warp to the extent seen in rickets. From the seventeenth through the nineteenth centuries many observers noted that rickets tended to occur in undernourished children living in the industrialized regions of Great Britain. It is a disease that occurred, and still occurs, though rarely, as a result of the conditions caused by industrialization in advanced civilizations.

Progress in uncovering the cause of the illness was slow, but gradually it was appreciated that both dietary and environmental factors are important in the etiology of rickets. The observation that cod liver oil produced marked improvement in children with rickets led to the hypothesis that the disease resulted from a paucity of fat in the diet. Then, in 1919, several important experiments were published by Edward Mellanby in England and K. Huldshinsky in Germany; these opened up a new era in understanding the cause of rickets and osteomalacia. Mellanby produced rickets in a group of young dogs by placing them on a series of diets composed primarily of milk and

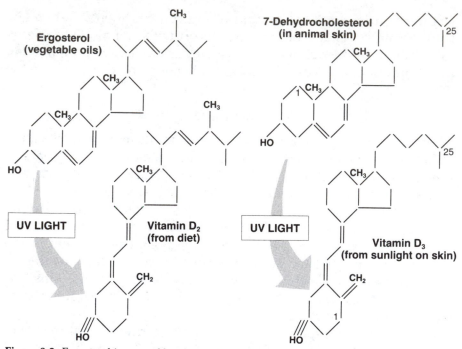

Figure 9-2. Ergosterol in vegetable oils and 7-dehydrocholesterol in animal skin are both converted into vitamin D by ultraviolet (UV) light. Vitamin D_2 is the primary source of vitamin D in the diet, whereas vitamin D_3 is produced within the body by skin exposed to sunlight.

carbohydrates. He was able to prevent rickets in some of the dogs by adding various vegetable and animal fats to the diets. These experiments demonstrated that diet plays an important role in preventing rickets. Animal fats, particularly cod liver oil, were most effective in preventing rickets, while vegetable oils varied widely in their effectiveness. Huldshinsky showed that rickets could be cured by exposing patients to sunlight or ultraviolet radiation irrespective of their diets. Thus, by the early 1920s, it was established that either a diet rich in animal fats *or* exposure to ultraviolet light could prevent or cure rickets, and the search was on for the antirachitic (anti-rickets) factor produced by these dual sources.

Two antirachitic factors were identified during the 1930s and designated vitamin D_2 and vitamin D_3 (see Figure 9-2). Because their chemical structures and biological action in humans are nearly identical, these vitamins are commonly referred to as vitamin D. Vitamin D_2 was the first antirachitic factor to be identified. When the plant substance called ergosterol is irradiated with ultraviolet light, it is converted into vitamin D_2. The discovery of this chemical reaction has allowed a simple preparation of vitamin D to be used in supplementing milk and other foodstuffs. Vitamin D_2 is also added to various vitamin preparations as a source of vitamin D. The widespread use of vitamin D_2 in foods and vitamin pills has nearly eliminated rickets as a disease entity, but cases do still occur, primarily in regions stricken by poverty.

In humans and other animals vitamin D_3 is produced in the skin from the precursor 7-dehydrocholesterol. The chemical reaction is a two-step affair, beginning with the rapid conversion of the precursor, by sunlight or ultraviolet radiation, to a compound called previtamin D_3, which is converted more slowly by heat to vitamin D_3. This reaction looks suspiciously like those we have seen in the synthesis of steroid hormones, where cholesterol-like precursors are converted by a series of chemical reactions to hormones such as cortisol and testosterone. After its synthesis in the skin, vitamin D_3 is released into the bloodstream, where it circulates, like the steroid hormones, bound to a carrier protein, in this case called vitamin D-binding protein (DBP). No vitamin D is necessary in the diet when there is ample exposure to sunlight, because the skin can synthesize what is required. In this sense vitamin D_3 is a hormone rather than a vitamin, because it is released into the circulation from the skin and is not required, as other vitamins are, in the diet—except when there is no sunlight exposure. This explains why rickets can occur only under conditions where there is too little sunlight coupled with a lack of vitamin D in the diet.

How does vitamin D act to insure an adequate calcification of bone and to help maintain a normal serum calcium level? Before the discovery of vitamin D, it was observed that children with rickets had a very high loss of dietary calcium into the feces, suggesting that cod liver oil or ultraviolet radiation cured rickets by somehow increasing the absorption of calcium in the intestine. This idea lay dormant until after vitamin D was isolated and available for studies in animals. A series of experiments in rats (by Nicolaysen and his colleagues in the late 1930s) established beyond doubt that one of the major actions of vitamin D is to increase the intestinal absorption of dietary calcium. It was naturally assumed that vitamin D itself was responsible for increasing the transport of calcium across the intestinal wall. This idea prevailed until the 1970s, when the remarkable discovery was made that it is *not* vitamin D at all that increases calcium transport from the gut but rather a metabolic product of vitamin D. With the discovery of a vitamin-D-dependent calcium-binding protein in the wall of the

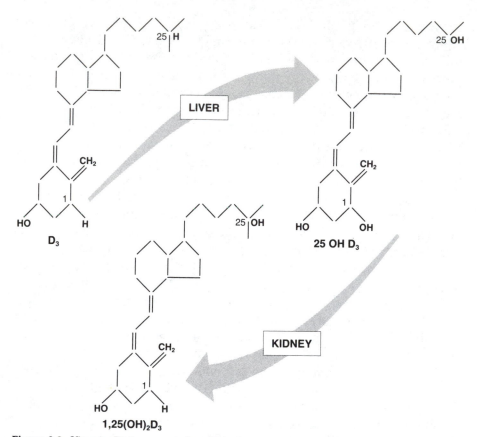

Figure 9-3. Vitamin D_3 is converted to 25 hydroxyvitamin D_3 in the liver and then to 1,25 dihydroxyvitamin D_3 in the kidneys by specific enzymes. The final metabolite $1,25(OH)_2D_3$ is the active form of vitamin D.

upper intestine, a comprehensive theory of vitamin D action became possible.

A key step in the discovery of biologically active vitamin D metabolite was the synthesis of radioactive preparations of D_2 and D_3. This enabled investigators to follow the metabolism of vitamin D into two important derivatives (see Figure 9-3). The first derivative to be discovered was 25-hydroxyvitamin D_3, which is made from circulating D_3 in the liver. The second important derivative is 1,25-hydroxyvitamin D_3, which is produced in the kidney. This derivative can actually be viewed as a hormone whose synthesis begins with 7-hydroxycholesterol, which is converted by sunlight-exposed skin to vitamin D_3, with subsequent modifications in the liver and kidneys.

How does the hormone 1,25-dihydroxyvitamin D_3 regulate calcium metabolism? It does so by binding to receptors in cells of the intestine and thereby promotes the synthesis of calcium-binding protein, which in turn transports calcium from the intestine into the circulation. By mechanisms that have not yet been defined it also promotes mobilization of calcium from the bones into the circulation. When 1,25-dihydroxyvitamin D_3 is deficient or does not work at its target sites, the serum calcium level falls below normal, because calcium is absorbed poorly from the diet and is not mobilized adequately from the bones. The low serum calcium level leads to an increase in serum PTH, resulting in an increased loss of phosphate into the urine and a lowered serum phosphate level. When the serum phosphate and calcium levels are low, newly forming bone is poorly mineralized; this results in rickets in children and in osteomalacia in adults.

Parathyroid Hormone

The discovery of the parathyroid glands in the late nineteenth century, followed by the demonstration that removal of the glands results in a low serum calcium level with consequent tetany, laid the foundation for the eventual isolation of parathyroid hormone by Collip in the mid-1920s. At this time the clinical syndrome of hyperparathyroidism had just been defined in Albert and Captain Martell, who were both cured of their disorder by removal of a PTH-secreting parathyroid tumor. In the 1940s, Fuller Albright and his colleagues at the Massachusetts General Hospital in Boston decribed a remarkable new syndrome in which patients were resistant to the action of parathyroid hormone. The PTH simply did not work and patients developed low levels of serum calcium with symptoms of tetany.

This was the first report in humans of a disorder where target sites were resistant to hormone action, although the reason for the resistance was not known at the time. Only much later did the concept of receptors evolve—a concept that hormones bind to receptors at target cells, initiating a series of metabolic events inside the cells.

The main function of parathyroid hormone is to regulate the serum calcium level within narrow limits, so that cells throughout the body will be bathed in extracellular fluid with just the right calcium concentration to support the proper functioning of the cells. Parathyroid hormone acts at two primary sites to perform this vital function—the bones and the kidneys. The osteoclast cells in bone are stimulated by PTH to resorb bone, releasing calcium into the circulation. Simultaneously, PTH acts on kidney tubule cells to resorb filtered calcium back into the bloodstream and prevent the loss of calcium in the urine. PTH also promotes the synthesis of 1,25-dihydroxyvitamin D from 25-hydroxyvitamin D in kidney cells, which leads to an increased absorption of calcium from the intestine. Therefore, by its direct action on bone and kidney cells, and by its indirect promotion of calcium absorption from the diet, parathyroid hormone is a critical factor in the maintenance of a normal serum calcium concentration.

The key signal for release of PTH from the parathyroid glands into the circulation is a falling serum calcium level, and conversely PTH release is diminished when the serum calcium concentration rises. The mechanism by which the serum calcium concentration controls the synthesis and release of PTH from parathyroid cells is not yet known, but this highly sensitive feedback system is perfectly honed to keep the serum calcium level where it belongs.

The synthesis of parathyroid hormone inside of the parathyroid cells is an elaborate affair and begins with synthesis of a 115-amino-acid precursor called pre-pro-PTH, which in turn is converted within seconds to the 90-amino-acid precursor pro-PTH. Finally, pro-PTH is converted into PTH, which is packaged into secretory granules awaiting release into the circulation when the serum calcium level falls. The whole process is shown in Figure 2-4, which depicts in schematic form the release of the 84-amino-acid PTH molecule into the circulation, where it is distributed to its target cells in the bone and kidney. The discovery of this intricate synthetic pathway has taken years of research in a number of different laboratories.

Parathyroid hormone stands at the center of a finely tuned metabolic system that tightly controls the serum calcium level. Not only does PTH regulate the flow of calcium between bone and serum, but it also prevents calcium loss in the urine and promotes the conversion of vitamin D to its active metabolite. When vitamin D or PTH is out of balance, disorders such as rickets, osteomalacia, hyperparathyroidism, or tetany can result. Thanks to scientific advances during this century, all of these disorders can now often be diagnosed and treated successfully. This is just one more example of the dramatic progress that has occurred in the field of hormone research.

10

THE NEUROPEPTIDE REVOLUTION

■

There's nothin' out there but computers—as far as the eye can see.
—Anonymous jogger, Stanford foothills, 1985

Not long ago I was standing at the top of one of the hills behind the Stanford Unversity campus, looking out across the Santa Clara valley toward San Jose. A jogger ran by, mumbled the words above, and then disappeared down the hill. He came complete with headband and the latest high tech jogging shoes, and generally gave the impression that he knew what he was talking about. I pondered his statement: Was he referring only to the Silicon Valley industries, or was he also referring to the people? The notion that we might be "nothin' but computers" left me with a rather uneasy feeling. And yet the neuropeptide revolution in brain chemistry and hormone physiology that has recently exploded does press in on our thoughts about freedom of choice and will.

I prefer to believe that a deeper understanding of how hormones and neurotransmitters work will not necessarily constrict our view of free will and lead us down a path of unyielding biological determinism. Rather such knowledge may very well expand our thinking about individual freedoms and serve as a basis for treating disorders of the mind and body that repress these freedoms.

We have finally come full circle. Starting in the first chapter with the evolution of peptide messengers, which were selected from an array of chemical structures in primitive organisms to be used as hormones in higher organisms, we now arrive at the extraordinary discovery of

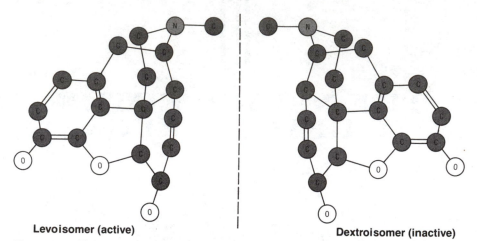

Levoisomer (active) **Dextroisomer (inactive)**

Figure 10-1. The two mirror-image forms of morphine are called stereoisomers. Even though these isomers are identical in composition, only the levo isomer is active as a narcotic.

peptide messengers in the brain and elsewhere throughout the nervous system. These small inconspicuous molecules, consisting of amino acids strung together in a linear chain, may ultimately prove to be important regulators of pain perception, temperature, appetite, intellect, and a variety of emotional states.

The use of opium as a medicine to relieve pain and as a euphoria-producing drug goes back to ancient Greece; indeed, the word opium comes from the Greek *opion*, meaning "poppy juice." Early in the nineteenth century opium was discovered to contain the alkaloid morphine. Morphine exists in two different mirror-image forms, called stereoisomers; they are levomorphine and dextromorphine (see Figure 10-1). To get an idea of how similar these stereoisomers really are, consider the following perturbation in your daily routine: When you straggle into the bathroom early one morning to bring yourself to life with a dash of cold water to the brow, take a hard look in the mirror. Set aside that usual narcissistic twinge of horror at recognizing that you are being ground down by the passage of time and take stock of the image. You are standing face to face with your stereoisomer—an image that looks very much like you except everything is turned around backward. The image's left hand is your right hand, and so on. In the case of morphine, the levoisomer is the active substance, producing euphoria and pain relief, while the dextroisomer is completely inactive. How could two molecules that are nearly identical in structure be so different in activity? This question led investigators to conclude that the brain contains highly specific receptors for the levoisomer of morphine and other morphine-like narcotics—receptors that could recognize levoisomers but not mirror-image dextroisomers. As we shall see, the pursuit of these stereospecific receptors opened a Pandora's box of knowledge about the action of morphine-like substances (the opioids) and ultimately led to the neuropeptide revolution.

The Search for Narcotic Receptors

On the surface of it, opioid receptors in animal brains should be easy to identify. Radiolabeled morphine derivatives can be prepared and then incubated with homogenates of brain tissues. Binding of the radiolabeled derivatives to opioid receptors present in the brain homogenates can then be measured in a radioactivity counter. The problem, however, with this type of experiment is that morphine binds loosely to many different nonspecific sites in brain tissue, and this nonspecific binding swamps out the binding to highly specific opioid receptors.

The first important attempt to circumvent this obstacle came in 1971 from the laboratory of Avram Goldstein at Stanford University School of Medicine. Goldstein reasoned that stereospecific opioid receptor binding could be determined for a radiolabeled morphine derivative, levorphanol, by subtracting out the nonspecific binding from the total binding. He homogenized brains from mice and prepared various subfractions of the homogenate by centrifugation techniques. He next measured the total binding of radiolabeled opiate (levorphanol labeled with radioactivity) to the brain homogenates—binding that was substantial. Nonspecific binding was determined by a series of experiments involving the competition of radiolabeled opiate with its nonradiolabeled duplicate and its mirror image isomer for the various binding sites. In this way he was able to determine that 53 percent of the opiate binding was to nonspecific receptors, 45 percent was trapped in the brain homogenate, and only 2 percent was bound to specific receptors. This disappointingly low 2 percent stereospecific binding possibly represented the presence of opioid receptors, but such a determination could not be made from this type of experiment until the large background of nonspecific binding could be reduced. Goldstein's use of stereoisomers was nevertheless an important advance.

A major breakthrough came in 1973, when Candace Pert and Solomon Snyder at Johns Hopkins University School of Medicine conclu-

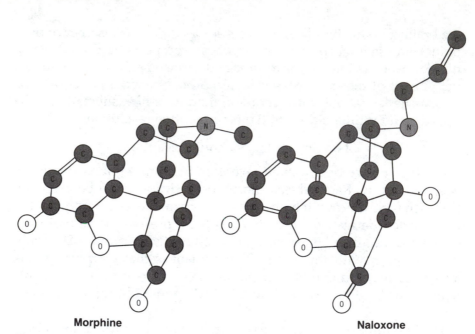

Morphine   **Naloxone**

Figure 10-2. Naloxone is a potent inhibitor of morphine. It is structurally similar to morphine and antagonizes the action of morphine by binding to opioid receptors.

sively demonstrated the existence of opioid receptors in rat brains and in nerve cells from guinea pig intestines. The success of their experiments hinged on two important technical innovations previously used by others in work on insulin receptors.

The first advance was to use an opioid compound labeled with a very high amount of radioactivity—they chose naloxone (see Figure 10-2); a potent antagonist of morphine, naloxone prevents morphine from binding to opioid receptors by directly competing for the receptors. The very high radioactivity allowed Pert and Snyder to use an extremely low concentration of naloxone, thus diminishing nonspecific binding while not sacrificing binding to high-affinity opioid receptors.

The second advance was to trap membrane fragments from homogenized brain cells onto filters, allowing very rapid washing—a maneuver that further reduced nonspecific binding. By these techniques they obtained a very high level of specific binding to homogenates from rat, mouse, and guinea pig brains—binding that was markedly diminished by excess levorphanol (morphine derivative) but not by its inactive stereoisomer dextrorphan. They also showed that excess amounts of many other morphine agonists (substances that act like morphine) inhibited naloxone binding, strongly supporting the notion that the radiolabeled naloxone was binding to opioid receptors.

Similar results were obtained with receptors isolated from the intestines of guinea pigs, where narcotics act to reduce the intensity of intestinal contractions. The link between opioid receptors in the intestine and opioid receptors in the brain proved to be critical in the eventual identification of the endogenous opioid peptides, those intriguing peptides made in the body that act at the same receptors as morphine.

Two other research groups, in Uppsala, Sweden, and in New York, also discovered opioid brain receptors in 1973, making it a banner year for investigations into the action of morphine and its derivatives. Taken together, these discoveries opened the way for the next important step in opioid research, the isolation of the body's own morphine-like chemicals that control pain perception and a variety of emotional states.

Discovery of the Enkephlins

With the demonstration that opioid receptors are present in the brain of many different animals, it was natural to wonder what they were doing there and to conjecture that they weren't simply there to interact with opium derivatives from poppy juice. That these receptors might be target sites for opium-like substances produced in the brain and perhaps elsewhere in the body was a much likelier hypothesis. Thus the search began for the hypothetical internal narcotics designated as *endogenous opioids*. Initial screens of homogenized brain extract for substances with the chemical characteristics of morphine-like alkaloids were unsuccessful, and the exploration broadened into a search through a wide range of different types of substances in brain extracts.

Success came when, in 1974, Lars Terenius and his co-workers at the University of Uppsala isolated from extracts derived from rat brains a factor that exhibited high-affinity binding to opioid receptors. Terenius had already independently isolated, from rat brain homogenates, opioid receptors that showed strong selective binding to a morphine derivative called dihydromorphine. He then began a search for the brain's own opioid substances by using this assay to screen extracts from homogenized rat brains. His initial attempts to isolate an endogenous brain factor that would bind tightly to the opioid receptors were unsuccessful because of improper extraction procedures. By diversifying his extraction methods he was finally able to isolate from rat brains a factor that does block dihydromorphine binding to opioid receptors. The purified factor is water soluble, is very low in molecular weight, and has chemical characteristics suggesting that it might be a small peptide. The same brain factor also blocks binding to opioid receptors extracted from guinea pig intestines.

Terenius was not alone in his discovery of an endogenous opioid factor. Simultaneously, John Hughes, Hans Kosterlitz, and their colleagues at the University of Aberdeen in Scotland were proceeding along a line of research that ultimately led them to a remarkable new discovery, the *enkephlins*. The enkephlins broke in on the world of brain research like a large wave crashing down on a novice surfer. Two small nondescript peptides, each only five amino acids long, the enkephlins are opioids produced in the brains of vertebrates, and they act like morphine at opioid receptors. These small peptides appear to be important in the regulation of pain pathways from peripheral nerves to the brain. They may also be important as inhibitors of muscle contractions in the intestines and elsewhere.

The starting point for the isolation of the enkephlins was a unique bioassay system for measuring the action of morphine and other opioid substances. Hughes and Kosterlitz prepared strips of muscle from guinea pig intestines and from the vas deferens of mice and stimulated them to contract by an electric signal. The contractions could be inhibited by low concentrations of opioids and thus could be used to test for the presence of endogenous opioids in brain extracts from pigs and other animals. The Aberdeen research team began by purifying extracts through a series of intricate chromatography steps, starting from a crude extract of 300 grams of pig brain. The purified extract showed marked inhibition of muscle contractions in the vas deferens assay, an inhibition that was completely reversed by the morphine antagonist naloxone. Similar results were obtained with the guinea pig intestine assay, but the extract had only about 20 percent of the activity seen in the vas deferens assay. They concluded that the brain extract contained an endogenous opioid acting at morphine receptors in the mouse vas deferens and guinea pig intestine, although the identity of this endogenous opioid had to await further investigation.

Others were closing in on endogenous opioids. Snyder at Johns Hopkins identified a morphine-like substance in calf and rat brains that displaced radiolabeled naloxone and dihydromorphine from opioid receptors—a substance that seemed chemically and physically similar to the factors isolated by Terenius and by Hughes and Koster-

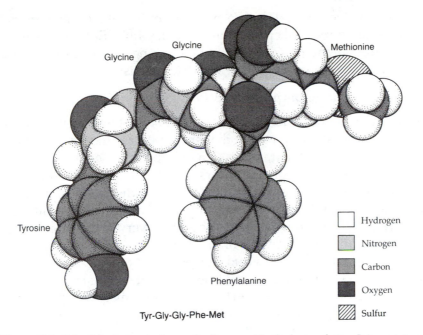

Glycine

Glycine

Methionine

	Hydrogen
	Nitrogen
	Carbon
	Oxygen
	Sulfur

Tyrosine

Phenylalanine

Tyr-Gly-Gly-Phe-Met

Figure 10-3. Enkephlin is a potent narcotic discovered in the brain of pigs. It is a pentapeptide composed of five amino acids strung together in a linear sequence. There are two different enkephlins: In met-enkephlin the fifth amino acid is methionine; in leu-enkephlin it is leucine.

litz. Meanwhile, Goldstein at Stanford extracted from the pituitary glands of cows a peptide that acted like morphine in several different assays but was larger than and chemically different from the other brain opioids.

The breakthrough by Hughes and Kosterlitz that launched the neuropeptide revolution was packed into a short, beautifully concise three-page paper entitled "Identification of Two Related Pentapeptides from the Brain with Potent Opiate Agonist Activity." This landmark paper, published in December 1975, describes how an extract from homogenized pig brains was carried through a detailed sequence of purification steps, then subjected to an amino acid analysis that showed the sequence of the first four amino acids to be tyrosine-glycine-glycine-phenylalanine, denoted as tyr-gly-gly-phe. Amino acid assignment to the fifth position was ambiguous, because the extract actually contained two peptides with different amino acids in the fifth position. The dilemma was resolved by subjecting the purified pig brain extract to mass spectrometric analysis, which suggested the presence of these two substances—one with the amino acid methionine in the fifth position (see Figure 10-3). The two new morphine-like brain peptides were designated met-enkephlin and leu-enkephlin. Both of these enkephlins are potent narcotic agonists showing about 20 times the activity of morphine in the mouse vas deferens assay.

The Endorphins and Pituitary Opioids

A revolutionary new view of the brain followed the discovery of the enkephlins. It was now apparent that small peptide molecules may be intimately involved in the transmission of important nerve signals and may themselves be neurotransmitters released at synaptic junctions between nerves. This new view has led to the discovery of a bewildering array of peptides other than opioids, both in the brain and elsewhere in the nervous system—peptides everywhere, completely overturning traditional views of brain chemistry.

The story of the *endorphins* and the pituitary opioids starts where the enkephlins left off. Hughes and Kosterlitz noticed that the 5-amino-acid sequence of met-enkephlin (tyr-gly-gly-phe-met) was present in the much larger 91-amino-acid peptide β-lipotropin, an unusual pituitary peptide discovered by C. H. Li at Berkeley in 1964, that still has no known function. It is a rather mysterious peptide, just standing around in the pituitary looking for something to do, but it is extraordinarily important because it stands at the crossroads between the enkephlins and the next group of endogenous opioids to be discovered, the *endorphins*, which are derived from it. Li stumbled across β-lipotropin while attempting to isolate ACTH from sheep pituitary glands, and eventually β-lipotropin was shown in humans, sheep, and other species to be a peptide composed of 91 amino acids. What is it doing there in the pituitary gland with so many other distinguished hormones?

A series of observations by several different research groups followed, demonstrating that β-lipotropin can give rise to a number of different peptides, all of which exhibit potent morphine-like activity in various opioid assays. These opioid peptides are called the endorphins, and all of them can be either isolated directly from the pituitary gland or produced by incubating β-lipotropin with brain extracts. Thus the function of β-lipotropin may simply be to serve as a precursor for the endorphins, rather than to perform a direct action itself.

After the discovery of the endorphins, a single very large pituitary peptide called pro-opiomelanocortin (POMC) was identified and found to contain the sequence for ACTH, β-lipotropin, and several other

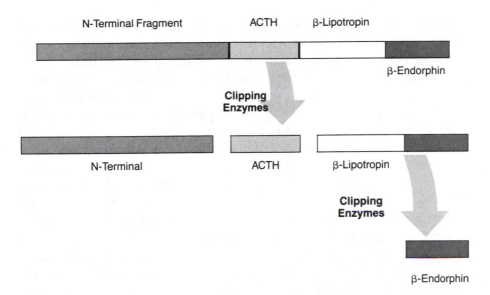

Figure 10-4. The large precursor peptide called pro-opiomelanocortin (POMC) contains the sequence for a number of peptides including ACTH and β-lipotropin. The anterior lobe of the pituitary gland contains enzymes which process POMC into smaller peptides.

peptides (see Figure 10-4). During stress, not only is increased ACTH released from the pituitary cells containing POMC, but β-lipotropin and β-endorphin are also released in increased amounts. ACTH, of course, promotes cortisol secretion by the adrenal glands, but the role of β-lipotropin and the opioid peptide β-endorphin during stress remains unknown. Certainly, nature must have something up its sleeve in creating these two interesting peptides, but so far no definite function has been uncovered. It seems highly unlikely that the gene for POMC would be conserved through evolutionary time without a role for any of its component peptides other than ACTH.

While the structures of the enkephlins and the endorphins were being unraveled, Goldstein and his colleagues at Stanford were struggling with the identity of a new, very potent opioid peptide they had discovered in extracts from pig pituitary glands in 1975. The new peptide proved to be extremely difficult to purify in large enough quantities to allow a chemical identification. But in 1979 an improvement in peptide sequencing techniques gave rise to the identification of dynorphin, a pituitary peptide nearly 1,000 times more potent than leu-enkephlin. Ultimately, dynorphin was shown to contain 17 amino acids, including the sequence for leu-enkephlin at its amino terminal end. Dynorphin is the most potent opioid peptide thus far isolated from animal brains and is widely distributed throughout the central nervous system as well as in the pituitary gland and the gut.

The role of these intriguing opioid peptides in the regulation of brain and body function is not yet known, but the chances are they will turn out to be important in the control of pain pathways and emotional states. Pain relief mechanisms such as acupuncture or placebos could very well be mediated in part by the endogenous opioid peptides. Regions of the central nervous system where electrical stimulation produces analgesia seem to have a high concentration of opioid receptors as well as endorphins or enkephlins, and each of the endogenous opioid peptides appears to have a unique distribution throughout the nervous system and to act at a number of different types of opioid receptors. Intravenous injections of the opioid peptides in humans produce characteristic alterations in the secretion of such pituitary hormones as ACTH, LH, FSH, prolactin, and growth hormone, while injections into the various ventricles of the brain produce pain relief. In spite of these interesting observations, we do not yet have a firm understanding of the role of the opioid peptides in the regulation of brain function.

Brain Peptides Galore

The isolation of the hypothalamic peptides TRH, LHRH, and somatostatin, followed by isolation of the endogenous opioid peptides, opened up a whole new vision of chemical messengers in the brain. Until these revolutionary discoveries we had a rather limited view of the types of messengers that are synthesized in nerve cells and then used to transmit regulatory signals to neighboring cells. The classical neurotransmitters are a small collection of such substances as acetylcholine, norepinephrine, dopamine, and serotonin, easily produced in nerve cells from simple precursors by enzymatic reactions. These amines are stored in nerve endings and are released by electrical discharges to transmit nerve signals to adjacent nerve cells. Next came the discovery that such simple amino acids as glycine, γ-aminobutyric acid (GABA), and glutamic acid could also serve as neurotransmitters. Until the discovery of the neuropeptides threw the whole classical concept into a fundamental upheaval, this handful of amines and amino acids were considered the basis of nerve cell signal transmission in the brain and elsewhere in the nervous system.

When sensitive antibody and chemical staining techniques were developed to detect the presence of hypothalamic and opioid peptides, it became possible to trace these substances in unsuspected regions of the nervous system and elsewhere throughout the body. The first nerve cells discovered to make peptides were the hypothalamic neurons that produce vasopressin and oxytocin. These peptides are synthesized in the cell bodies of large neurons located in the hypothalamus. They are then packaged into granules, transported down the nerve cell axon to the posterior pituitary gland, and stored until they are released into the general circulation; vasopressin acts at the kidney to conserve water, and oxytocin acts to induce contractions in the uterus. It has recently been discovered, surprisingly, that some of the hypothalamic neurons containing vasopressin send their axons into the central nervous system, where they terminate in the thalamus and other structures of the brain stem and spinal cord. Thus, the peptide vasopressin can function as a hormone when the axons terminate in the posterior pituitary and as a neurotransmitter when the axons terminate on other nerve cells in the brain or spinal cord. Nature has chosen to use the same peptide to operate in both communication systems.

The hypothalamus is the site of other peptide-producing nerve cells besides those that make vasopressin and oxytocin. All of the hypothalamic peptides regulating anterior pituitary hormone secretion are produced in nerve cell bodies located in various regions of the hypothalamus. These peptides are released from nerve cell axon endings into the portal circulation in the upper region of the pituitary stalk and are transported to the anterior pituitary, where they interact with cells that make the pituitary hormones ACTH, TSH, LH, FSH, growth hormone, and prolactin.

The isolation of TRH, the first hypothalamic-releasing hormone isolated by Schally and Guillemin, was one of the key events that catapulted us into the neuropeptide revolution. But the book was not closed on TRH with this exciting discovery; new sensitive assay techniques reveal TRH not only in nerve cells in the hypothalamus but in neurons throughout the brain as well. About 80 percent of the TRH in the brain of a rat is located outside of the hypothalamus—and receptors for TRH are also scattered throughout the same regions of the brain. What looked on the surface of things like a simple peptide, manufactured in neurons of the hypothalamus in order to regulate release of TSH from the pituitary, has turned out on deeper probing to be a much more complex factor. The TRH scattered throughout the brain undoubtedly functions as a neurotransmitter in a variety of brain neurons, possibly regulating appetite and various mood states, although at present its specific function in the brain remains a mystery. TRH is one of several peptides with a dual function—as a hormone to regulate pituitary cells and as a neurotransmitter elsewhere in the brain.

The discovery of somatostatin by Guillemin and his colleagues was pivotal in firmly establishing the theory of pituitary function regulation by hormones from the hypothalamus. At the time of its initial discovery, no one would have guessed in their wildest speculations that somatostatin would turn out to be a ubiquitous chemical messenger, scattered all over the body and in the most diverse locations—a peptide for all seasons. Somatostatin, the 14-amino-acid peptide synthesized in hypothalamic neurons, suppresses growth hormone release from cells in the anterior pituitary. It is not only located in neurons throughout the brain, where it most likely functions in the transmission of nerve signals, but it is also found in sensory nerves of the spinal cord; in the stomach and intestines, where it inhibits gastrin secretion; and in the pancreas, where it inhibits the secretion of insulin and glucagon. In the hypothalamus it acts as a hormone to inhibit growth hormone secretion from the pituitary gland; in the nervous system it acts as a neurotransmitter; and in the pancreas it directly inhibits hormone secretion from neighboring alpha and beta cells. By enabling it to perform endocrine, neurotransmitter, and paracrine functions, evolution has contrived to use somatostatin for a broad array of regulatory purposes.

There is an economy here in the extraordinary union of the endocrine and nervous systems—control networks that were initially thought to be entirely independent of each other. The enkephlins and their corresponding opioid receptors are widely distributed throughout the brain, spinal cord, and intestines. As one might expect, since the enkephlins are endogenous opioids, nerve cells containing enkephlin seem to be particularly prevalent in regions of the nervous system associated with pain perception. The neurons that utilize enkephlins as neurotransmitters inhibit nerve cells responsible for the conduction of pain sensation from the original pain receptors to the spinal cord and the brain. Similar enkephlin nerve tracts are found in regions of the brain responsible for mood and in regions of the brain stem that regulate respiration. Enkephlin-containing nerve cells are also located in the intestines, where they appear to control muscle contractions.

TABLE 10-1

Peptides Found in Both the Brain and the Intestines

Bombesin
Cholecystokinin Octapeptide (CCK-8)
Glucagon
Insulin
Leu-Enkephlin
Met-Enkephlin
Neurotensin
Substance P
Vasoactive Intestinal Polypeptide (VIP)

These observations correlate with long-standing clinical observations that morphine and other opioid-like drugs can simultaneously relieve pain, produce euphoria, suppress respiration, and give rise to severe constipation.

Somatostatin and the enkephlins are not the only peptides in both the brain and intestines acting as neurotransmitters or hormones. A whole series of peptides have been discovered to reside in both places (see Table 10-1). These peptides have exotic designations like substance P, bombesin, VIP, neurotensin, and CCK-8, and are undoubtedly only the first wave of a much larger assortment of peptides yet to be uncovered. Some investigators estimate that the number of peptides in the brain acting as neurotransmitters may approximate 200. Whatever the number eventually turns out to be, it will certainly be much larger than the presently identified 20 to 30 peptides.

Von Euler and Gaddum, during their investigation of the distribution of acetylcholine in various tissues of horses, found a new compound, primarily in the brain and intestines of the horses, that stimulated intestinal contractions and produced a fall of blood pressure in rabbits. Forty years later this substance P was isolated in pure form and shown to be a peptide containing 11 amino acids. Present in neurons distributed widely throughout the peripheral and central nervous system, it seems to be closely associated with nerve pathways regulating pain perception and emotional behavior.

Neurotensin shows a distribution similar to enkephlin and substance P. Initially isolated in 1973 during the course of a purification procedure for substance P, neurotensin is a peptide, containing 13 amino acids, that lowers blood pressure in rats and stimulates contractions in preparations of guinea pig intestines. The distribution of neurotensin throughout the brain is strikingly similar to the distribution of enkephlin, although the two peptides appear to be located in different neurons. The decrease in pain perception induced by neurotensin is not blocked by the opioid antagonist naloxone, implying that neurotensin acts through its own receptors in pain pathways rather than through opioid receptors. In spite of its being like enkephlin and substance P, located throughout the nervous system, neurotensin remains a peptide whose function is not yet fully understood.

Several peptides originally discovered in the small intestine, and identified as hormones regulating functions related to the digestion of foods, have more recently been discovered in the brain. Vasoactive intestinal polypeptide (VIP) is a 28-amino-acid peptide (first isolated in 1970) remarkably similar in structure to secretin and glucagon. VIP has a broad range of biological actions, including the lowering of blood pressure by dilation of arterioles, the increased production of glucose from glycogen, the stimulation of secretions by the intestines and pancreas, and the inhibition of gastric acid secretion by the stomach. VIP has been found throughout the gastrointestinal tract from the esophagus to the rectum. Recently it has been discovered in neurons of the brain, primarily in the cerebral cortex, where it appears to activate the vertically oriented columns of nerves in the outer cortex. Thus, in addition to its role as a hormone in regulating blood pressure and intestinal function, VIP appears to serve as a neurotransmitter in the higher cortical regions of the brain.

Cholecystokinin (CCK) is another peptide hormone initially isolated from the small intestine and later shown to be found in the brain. It contains a sequence of 33 amino acids and derives its name from the fact that it stimulates contractions of the gall bladder. It is a hormone designed to promote digestion by stimulating the pancreas to release bile and pancreatic juices into the small intestine. Although CCK produced by intestinal-lining cells is 33 amino acids long, the peptide with CCK activity found in the brain is almost exclusively CCK-8 (the 8-amino-acid sequence contained in the carboxyl-terminal end of CCK-33). There is a widespread distribution of CCK-8 throughout the nervous system, including the cerebral cortex, the hypothalamus, the brain stem, and sensory nerves in the spinal cord. It appears to be the only brain peptide (along with VIP) in the cerebral cortex, where it exerts a potent excitation of cortical neurons. There is some evidence that in animals CCK-8 may be an important regulator of feeding behavior.

Bombesin is a 14-amino-acid peptide originally isolated from skin of the European frog *Bombina bombina*, an unlikely source of a mammalian neuropeptide. However, bombesin is known to stimulate gastric acid secretion, gall bladder contraction, and pancreatic enzyme secretion in different mammals. Intravenous infusion of bombesin in humans produces a rise in plasma insulin, glucagon, CCK, gastrin, and other hormones. Antibodies against bombesin have shown activity in the brain, the lungs, and the gastrointestinal tract. When injected into the brains of rats, bombesin produces a lowering of the body temperature. Thus bombesin (or peptides with structure similar to bombesin) appears to have widespread effects throughout the body, including the brain and intestines.

The neuropeptide revolution started quietly with the isolation of vasopressin and oxytocin, produced by nerve cells in the hypothalamus and stored in the posterior pituitary gland. The view broadened with the discovery of TRH, LHRH, and somatostatin—hypothalamic peptides that control synthesis of hormones in the anterior pituitary gland. And now, with the discovery of the enkephlins, the door is opening into the far reaches of the brain, where a variety of peptides have been identified as potential neurotransmitters. Although it was suspected that endogenous opioids such as the enkephlins would turn up in the brain, not even the most starry-eyed dreamer ever conjectured that peptides like bombesin, insulin, VIP, TRH, and CCK-8 would also be found scattered throughout the brain, defying conventional views of brain nerve cell physiology.

So here we are at last, inching toward a tentative understanding of this seemingly vast maze of chemical messengers. After working our way through a virtual jungle of hormones and neurotransmitters, we are ready to settle back, dust a few cobwebs off the neocortex, and briefly take stock of the whole picture.

Back in the days, eons ago, when total chaos reigned (some would say things are not much different today), life came struggling out of the sea of simple atoms and molecules in the form of single cells. Early on, chemical messengers arrived on the scene to enhance communication between cells, coordinating events to promote survival in a world where survival was in constant jeopardy. In the evolution of the chemical messengers from primitive organisms to humans, there has been an extraordinary conservation of valuable chemical structures in the form of peptides, shifting their way into the nooks and crannies of regulatory sites such as the higher brain, the hypothalamus and pituitary, the gastrointestinal tract, and undoubtedly many other as yet undisclosed locations.

These messengers of life didn't appear spontaneously out of nowhere. Rather, nature unfolded the messengers slowly, tinkering away through evolution, picking up useful scraps here and there, and stitching them into a harmoniously layered patchwork. Peptides in bacteria and other lower organisms gradually gave way to similar peptides in the endocrine glands and nervous systems of higher organisms. Simple signals gave way to complex signals as evolution hammered out its unique design. No one knows what evolution will produce in the future, but it is certain that whatever forms of beings are created will be etched out of today's scraps, slowly, without a concise blueprint.

At present, we can only hold our breath and continue the quest for knowledge of things as they exist now—a quest that will surely lead us to a deeper understanding of the mysterious workings of the human brain and, we hope, to more profound therapies for disorders of the brain that have afflicted us throughout recorded history. Imagine a world in which maladies like schizophrenia, psychotic depression, and Alzheimer's disease can be effectively treated! There is, then, in this astounding labyrinth of chemical messengers, a certain hope for the future—if we can only rise to the adventure and press forward with the exciting research tasks at hand.

BIBLIOGRAPHY

Chapter 1

Bayliss, W. M., and E. H. Starling. "The Mechanism of Pancreatic Secretion." *Journal of Physiology (London)* 28 (1902): 325-53.

Dickerson, R. E. "Chemical Evolution and the Origin of Life." *Scientific American* 239 (1978): 70-86.

Jacob, F. "Evolution and Tinkering." *Science* 196 (1977): 1161-66.

Martin, C. J. "Ernest Henry Starling—Life and Work." *British Medical Journal* 1 (1927): 900-904.

Medvei, V. C. *A History of Endocrinology.* Lancaster, England: MTP Press, 1982. (This reference has been used throughout the book as a source of historical information.)

Roth, J., D. LeRoith, J. Shiloach, et al. "The Evolutionary Origins of Hormones, Neurotransmitters, and Other Extracellular Chemical Messengers." *New England Journal of Medicine* 306 (1982): 523-27.

Schaefer, E. A. "Internal Secretions." *Lancet* 2 (1895): 321-24.

Starling, E. H. "The Chemical Correlation of the Functions of the Body." *Lancet* 2 (1905): 339-41.

Sutherland, E. W. "Studies on the Mechanism of Hormone Action." *Science* 177 (1972): 401-8.

Thomas, L. *The Lives of a Cell: Notes of a Biology Watcher*, 17-21. New York: Bantam Books, 1975.

Wilson, E. O. "Pheromones." *Scientific American* 208 (1963): 100-114.

Yalow, R. S. "Radioimmunoassay: A Probe for the Fine Structure of Biologic Systems." *Science* 200 (1978): 1236-45.

Chapter 2

Catt, K. J., and M. L. Dufau. "Hormone Action: Control of Target-Cell Function by Peptide, Thyroid, and Steroid Hormones." In *Endocrinology and Metabolism*, eds. P. Felig, J. D. Baxter, A. E. Broadus, et al., 61-105. San Francisco: McGraw-Hill, 1981.

Federman, D. D. "General Principles of Endocrinology." In *Textbook of Endocrinology*, ed. R. H. Williams, 1-14. Philadephia: W. B. Saunders Company, 1981.

Habener, J. F. "Hormone Biosynthesis and Secretion." In *Endocrinology and Metabolism*, eds. P. Felig, J. D. Baxter, A. E. Broadus, et al., 29-59. San Francisco: McGraw Hill, 1981.

Roth, J., and C. Grunfeld. "Endocrine Systems: Mechanisms of Disease, Target Cells, and Receptors." In *Textbook of Endocrinology*, ed. R. H. Williams, 15-72. Philadelphia: W. B. Saunders Company, 1981.

Chapter 3

Guillemin, R., P. Brazeau, P. Bohlen, et al. "Growth Hormone-Releasing Factor from a Human Pancreatic Tumor that Caused Acromegaly." *Science* 218 (1982): 585-87.

Guillemin, R., and R. Burgus. "The Hormones of the Hypothalamus." *Scientific American* 227 (1972): 24-33.

Harris, G. W. "Humours and Hormones." *Journal of Endocrinology* 53 (1972): ii-xxii.

————. *Neural Control of the Pituitary Gland*. London: Edward Arnold Publishers, 1955.

Krieger, D. T., and J. C. Hughes, eds. *Neuroendocrinology*. Sutherland, Massachusetts: Sinauer Associates Inc., 1980.

Meites, J., B. T. Donovan, and S. M. McCann, eds. *Pioneers in Neuroendocrinology*. New York: Plenum Press, 1965. (This book contains a number of short articles about regulation of the pituitary by the hypothalamus written by a number of the scientists involved in the pioneering research, including Schally and Guillemin.)

Rivier, J., J. Spiess, M. Thorner, et al. "Characterization of a Growth Hormone-Releasing Factor from a Human Pancreatic Islet Tumor." *Nature* 300 (1982): 276-78.

Schally, A. V., A. Arimura, and A. J. Kastin. "Hypothalamic Regulatory Hormones." *Science* 179 (1973): 341-50.

Vale, W., J. Spiess, C. Rivier, et al. "Characterization of a 41 Residue Ovine Hypothalamic Peptide that Stimulates Secretion of Corticotropin and β-Endorphin." *Science* 213 (1981): 1394-97.

Wade, N. *The Nobel Duel: Two Scientists' 21-Year Race to Win the World's Most Coveted Research Prize*. Garden City, New York: Anchor Press, Doubleday, 1981. (An exciting book about the race between Schally and Guillemin to discover the structure of hypothalamic hormones. I have drawn heavily on it as a reference for behind-the-scenes details of this tremendous research effort.)

Chapter 4

Brownstein, M. J., J. T. Russell, and H. Gainer. "Synthesis, Transport, and Release of Posterior Pituitary Hormones." *Science* 207 (1980): 373-78.

Greep, R. O. "History of Research on Anterior Hypophysial Hormones." In *Handbook of Physiology*, exec. ed. S. R. Geiger, Section 7, *Endocrinology*, eds. R. O. Greep and E. B. Astwood, vol. IV, *The Pituitary and Its Neuroendocrine Control*, eds. E. Knobil and W. H. Sawyer, part 2, 1-28. Washington, D. C.: American Physiological Society, 1974.

Heller, H. "History of Neurohypophysial Research." In *Handbook of Physiology*, Section 7, vol. IV, part 1, 103-18.

Major, R. H. *Classic Description of Disease*. 3rd ed. Springfield, Illinois: Charles C. Thomas Publisher, 1945.

Chapter 5

Cardinali, D. P. "Melatonin: A Mammalian Pineal Hormone." *Endocrine Reviews* 2 (1981): 327-46.

McCord, C. P., and F. P. Allen. "Evidences Associating Pineal Gland Function with Alterations in Pigmentation." *Journal of Experimental Zoology* 23 (1917): 207-24.

Neuwelt, E. A., and A. J. Lewy. "Disappearance of Plasma Melatonin after Removal of a Neoplastic Pineal Gland." *New England Journal of Medicine* 308 (1983): 1132-35.

Preslock, J. P. "The Pineal Gland: Basic Implications and Clinical Correlations." *Endocrine Reviews* 5 (1984): 282-308.

Reiter, R. J. "The Pineal and Its Hormones in the Control of Reproduction in Mammals." *Endocrine Reviews* 1 (1980): 109-31.

Wurtman, R. J. "The Pineal as a Neuroendocrine Transducer." *Hospital Practice* 15 (1980): 82-92.

Wurtman, R. J., and J. Axelrod. "The Pineal Gland." *Scientific American* 213 (1965): 2-12.

Wurtman, R. J., and M. A. Moskowitz. "The Pineal Organ." *New England Journal of Medicine* 296 (1977): 1329-33, 1383-86.

Chapter 6

Crawford, J. D. "It's a Boy?" *New England Journal of Medicine* 291 (1974): 976-77.

Federman, D. D. *Abnormal Sexual Development*. Philadelphia: W. B. Saunders Company, 1967.

———. "His and Hers." *New England Journal of Medicine* 290 (1974): 1137.

Haseltine, F P., and S. Ohno. "Mechanisms of Gonadal Determination and Gametogenesis." *Science* 211 (1981): 1272-78.

Imperato-McGinley, J., R. E. Peterson, T. Gautier, et al. "Androgens and the Evolution of Male-Gender Identity among Male Pseudohermaphrodites with 5α-Reductase Deficiency." *New England Journal of Medicine* 300 (1979): 1233-77.

Jost, A. "Problems of Fetal Endocrinology: The Gonadal and Hypophyseal Hormones." *Recent Progress in Hormone Research* 8 (1953): 379-418.

Levine, S. "Sexual Differentiation: The Development of Maleness and Femaleness." *Western Journal of Medicine* 114 (1971): 12-17.

Naftolin, F. "Understanding the Bases of Sex Differences." *Science* 211 (1981): 1263-64.

Wilson, J. D., F. W. George, and J. E. Griffin. "The Hormonal Control of Sexual Development." *Science* 211 (1981): 1278-84.

Wilson, J. D., J. E. Griffin, M. Leshin, et al. "The Androgen Resistance Syndromes: 5α-Reductase Deficiency, Testicular Feminization, and Related Disorders." In *The Metabolic Basis of Inherited Disease*, 5th ed., eds. J. B. Stanbury, J. B. Wyngaarden, D. S. Fredrickson, et al., 1001-26. San Francisco: McGraw-Hill, 1983.

Chapter 7

Bergland, R. M. "New Information Concerning the Irish Giant." *Journal of Neurosurgery* 23 (1965): 265-69.

Daughaday, W. H. "Extreme Gigantism." *New England Journal of Medicine* 297 (1977): 1267-69.

Friesen, H. G. "Raben Lecture 1980: A Tale of Stature." *Endocrine Reviews* 1 (1980): 309-18.

Hintz, R. L., D. M. Wilson, J. Finno, et al. "Biosynthetic Methionyl Human Growth Hormone Is Biologically Active in Adult Man." *Lancet* 1 (1982): 1276-79.

Laron, Z. "Syndrome of Familial Dwarfism and High Plasma Immunoreactive Growth Hormone." *Israel Journal of Medical Science* 10 (1974): 1247-53.

Marimee, T. J., J. Zapf, and E. R. Froesch. "Dwarfism in the Pigmy: An Isolated Deficiency of Insulin-Like Growth Factor I." *New England Journal of Medicine* 305 (1981): 965-68.

Phillips, L. S., and R. Vassilopoulou-Sellin. "Somatomedins." *New England Journal of Medicine* 302 (1980): 371-80, 438-44.

Rudman, D., M. H. Kutner, R. D. Blackston, et al. "Children with Normal-Variant Short Stature: Treatment with Human Growth Hormone for Six Months." *New England Journal of Medicine* 305 (1981): 123-31.

Van Wyk, J. J., and L. E. Underwood. "Growth Hormone, Somatomedins, and Growth Failure." *Hospital Practice* 13 (1978): 57-67.

Chapter 8

Bliss, M. *The Discovery of Insulin*. Chicago: University of Chicago Press, 1982.

Burrow, G. N., B. E. Hazlett, and M. J. Phillips. "A Case of Diabetes Mellitus." *New England Journal of Medicine* 306 (1982): 340-43.

Cahill, G. F. "Metabolic Fuels." *Anesthesia Analgesia Current Research* 44 (1965): 478-86.

———. "Starvation in Man." *New England Journal of Medicine* 282 (1970): 668-75.

Kerndt, P. R., J. L. Naughton, C. E. Driscoll, et al. "Fasting: The History, Pathophysiology, and Complications." *Western Journal of Medicine* 137 (1982): 379-99.

Medvei, V. C. *A History of Endocrinology*. Lancaster, England: MTP Press, 1982, 454-70.

Orci, L., and R. H. Unger. "Functional Subdivision of Islets of Langerhans and Possible Role for D Cells." *Lancet* 2 (1975): 1243-44.

Chapter 9

Albright, F. "A Page Out of the History of Hyperparathyroidism." *Journal of Clinical Endocrinology and Metabolism* 8 (1948): 637-57.

Baur, W., and D. D. Federman. "Hyperparathyroidism Epitomized: The Case of Captain Charles E. Martell." *Metabolism* 11 (1962): 21-29.

DeLuca, H. F. "The Vitamin D Hormonal System: Implications for Bone Diseases." *Hospital Practice* 15 (1980): 57-63.

Haussler, M. R., and T. A. McCain. "Basic and Clinical Concepts Related to Vitamin D Metabolism and Action." *New England Journal of Medicine* 297 (1977): 974-831, 1041-50.

Kodicek, E. "The Story of Vitamin D from Vitamin to Hormone." *Lancet* 1 (1974): 325-29.

Chapter 10

Goldstein, A. "Opioid Peptides (Endorphins) in Pituitary and Brain." *Science* 193 (1976): 1081-86.

Hughes, J., T. W. Smith, H. W. Kosterlitz, et al. "Identification of Two Related Pentapeptides from the Brain with Potent Opiate Agonist Activity." *Nature* 258 (1975): 577-79.

Kosterlitz, H. W., and A. T. McKnight. "Endorphins and Enkephlins." *Advances in Internal Medicine* 26 (1980): 1-36.

Krieger, D. T., and A. S. Liotta. "Pituitary Hormones: Where, How, Why?" *Science* 205 (1979): 366-72.

Krieger, D. T., and J. B. Martin. "Brain Peptides." *New England Journal of Medicine* 304 (1981): 876-85, 944-51.
Snyder, S. H. "Brain Peptides as Neurotransmitters." *Science* 209 (1980): 976-83.
———. "Opiate Receptors and Internal Narcotics." *Scientific American* 236 (1977): 44-56.
"Brain Peptides—New Synaptic Messengers?" *Lancet* 2 (1980): 895-96.
"Endogenous Opiates and Their Actions." *Lancet* 2 (1982): 305-7.

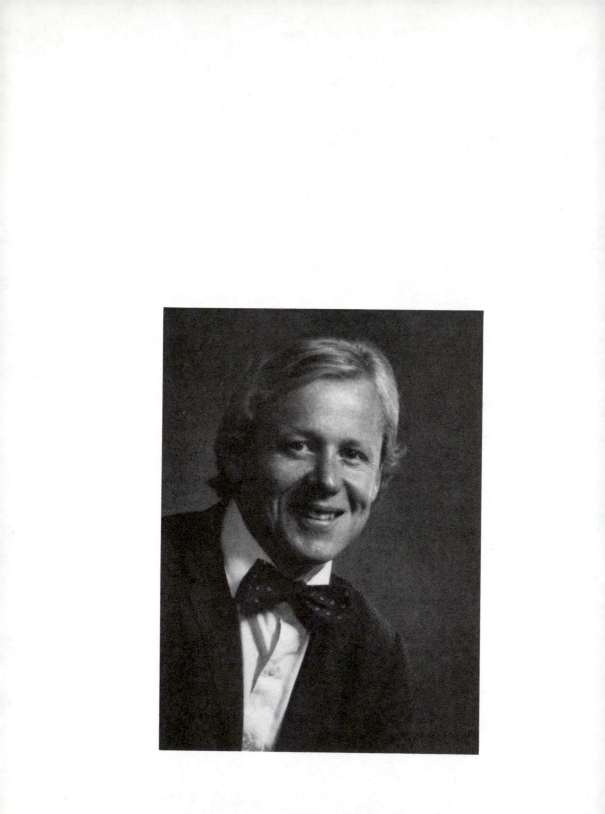

ABOUT THE AUTHOR

Lawrence Crapo is on the full-time faculty in the Department of Medicine at the Stanford University School of Medicine and is chief of endocrinology at the Santa Clara Valley Medical Center, a Stanford-affiliated county hospital in San Jose. In 1984 he was the recipient of a Kaiser Award for Excellence in Teaching Clinical Medicine at Stanford Medical School.

Dr. Crapo earned his bachelor of science degree in chemistry from the University of California at Berkeley and his Ph.D. from the physics department at Harvard, where he studied the nuclear magnetic resonance properties of small molecules in a high-vacuum molecular beam. He spent another three years at Harvard pursuing postdoctoral research in molecular biology in the laboratory of James Watson and Walter Gilbert, where he participated in investigations related to the regulation of the genetic code in bacteria.

After obtaining his M. D. at Stanford University School of Medicine and completing his residency in medicine at the Stanford Medical Center, Dr. Crapo returned to Boston as a fellow in endocrinology at the Massachusetts General Hospital, where he studied the mechanism of insulin action with Joseph Avruch. He has recently completed a research project on the complications of diabetic coma syndromes.

Dr. Crapo has published original papers in the fields of chemistry, physics, molecular biology, and medicine and is coauthor of a recent book on the biology of human aging, called *Vitality and Aging*. He presently lives on the Stanford University campus with his wife, two children, one Samoyed dog, one chinchilla rabbit, and two goldfish. His nonscientific passions include soccer, tennis, and modern jazz.

Series Editor: Miriam Miller
Production Manager: Laura Ackerman-Shaw
Book Design: Andrew Danish
Cover Design: Robin Hessel
Illustrations: Pamela Manley

CREDITS

The following material has been reproduced with the kind permission of the individuals and institutions listed.

Page
1   Quotation from F. Jacob, "Evolution and Tinkering," *Science* 196 (10 June 1977): 1146. Copyright 1977 by AAAS.
9   Quotation from C. J. Martin, "Ernest Henry Starling—Life and Work," *British Medical Journal* 1 (14 May 1927): 902.
17   Quotation from L. Thomas, *The Lives of a Cell*, New York: Bantam Books, 1977, page 18.
27   *Figure 2-3*. J. Haebner and J. Potts, "Biosynthesis of Parathyroid Hormone, I," *New England Journal of Medicine* 299 (14 September 1978): 582.
28   *Figure 2-4*. J. Haebner and J. Potts, "Biosynthesis of Parathyroid Hormone, II," *New England Journal of Medicine*, 299 (21 September 1978): 636.
65   *Akhenaten*. The National Museum at Berlin, DDR, Egyptian Museum, number 14 512.
67   *Dachshund Dogs*. H. Evans, et al., *The Growth and Gonad-Stimulating Hormones of the Anterior Hypophysis*, Memoirs of the University of California, vol. II. Berkeley, CA: University of California Press, 1933.
83   *Figure 5-4*. R. J. Wurtman, "The Effects of Light on the Human Body," *Scientific American* 233 (July 1975): 71.
87   *Figure 5-5*. R. Reiter, "The Pineal and Its Hormones in the Control of Reproduction in Mammals," *Endocrine Reviews* 1 (Spring 1980): 122.
91   *Figure 5-6*. E. Neuwelt and A. Lewy, "The Disappearance of Plasma Melatonin after Removal of a Neoplastic Pineal Gland," *New England Journal of Medicine* 308 (12 May 1983): 1134.
95   *Human Chromosomes*. Stanford Medical Center, Cytogenetics Laboratory.
99   *Figure 6-1*. J. E. Giffin and J. D. Wilson, "The Syndromes of Androgen Resistance," *New England Journal of Medicine* 302 (24 January 1980): 1278.
102 *Figure 6-2*. J. D. Wilson, et al., "The Hormonal Control of Sexual Development," *Science* 211 (20 March 1981): 1279. Copyright 1981 by AAAS.

INDEX

Brain tumors, 121
Brazeau, P., 54
Burgus, R., 44, 47-49, 50, 52, 54-55
Byrne, Charles, 116, 117-118

Calcium, 23, 28, 34, 147-160 passim
Castrates, 6, 100, 109
"Chemical Correlation of the Functions of the Body," 11
Chevreul, Michel-Eugène, 130
Cholecystokinin (CCK), 14, 23, 174
Cholesterol, 26, 31
Chromosomes, 93-108
Circulation, of diabetics, 145
Classical view, 13, 20, 25
Cod liver oil, for rickets, 155, 156
Collip, J. B., 76, 135, 151, 159
Congenital adrenal hyperplasia (CAH), 110
Cortex, adrenal, 24-25
Corticotropin-releasing hormone (CRH), 24-25, 42-44, 55-56
Cortisol, 24-25, 31-32, 75, 76, 103, 142
Cretinism, 72, 73
CRH, see Corticotropin-releasing hormone
C-terminal, 48, 50
Cushing, Harvey, 61, 66, 68, 117
Cyclic adenosine monophosphate (cyclic AMP), 11-12, 16, 30-31, 32, 56, 138
Cytoplasm, 29

Daughaday, W. H., 125, 127
7-dehydrocholesterol, 157
Deoxyribonucleic acid (DNA), 3-4, 6, 26, 96
Descartes, René, 79, 88
Deuben, R. R., 54, 56
Dextromorphine, 162
Diabetes insipidus, 61-62
Diabetes mellitus, 7, 23, 62, 129-136, 140, 143-146
    Type I, 144
    Type II, 144-145
Diabetic ketoacidosis, 143-144, 145
Digestion, 23-24
Dihydromorphine, 165-166
Dihydrotestosterone (DHT), 101, 104, 106-107
DNA, see Deoxyribonucleic acid

Dobson, Matthew, 130
Dominican Republic, 93-94, 101, 106, 110-111
DuBois, Eugene, 147-148
Dwarfs, 119-122, 123
Dynorphin, 23, 169-170

Education, science, 12
Endocrine function, of pancreas, 130
Endocrine systems, 4-7, 11, 12, 59
    classical view of, 13, 20, 25
    with nervous system, 4, 9, 15, 37-40, 172
Endocrinology, 8, 11, 12-13, 40
Endogenous opioids, 165-166, 172, 175
β-endorphin, 23, 76, 169-170
Endorphins, 168-170
Enkephlins, 165-168, 172, 174, 175
Enzmann, F., 50, 54
Enzymes, 16, 33, 107
Epinephrine, 8, 11, 25, 30, 33, 84, 142
Erdheim, Jacob, 150
Escherichia coli, 128
Estradiol, 25, 31, 69, 101, 105, 108, 109
Estrogen, 69, 105, 109
Euler, U.S. von, 173
Evans, Herbert M., 66, 68, 122-123
Evolution, 1-18, 176
Exocrine function, 130
External secretion, 7
Eye disease, diabetics and, 145, 146

Fasting, 140-142
Fat cells
    during fasting, 141-142
    insulin in, 140, 142
Fats, dietary, rickets and, 155, 156
Fawcett, Peter, 51
Female pseudohermaphrodites, 103
Fielding, Una, 40
Finland, 91
First messengers, 12, 31
Fiske, Virginia, 82
Folkers, K., 50, 54
Follicle-stimulating hormone (FSH), 37, 67-68, 69, 108-114 passim
    LHRH and, 50, 53, 68, 88, 108, 111
    pineal function and, 86, 88
Fröhlich, Alfred, 61, 68

Kappers, Ariëns, 82, 89
Keith, Arthur, 117
Ketoacidosis, 143, 144, 145
Ketones, 144
Kidney function
  of diabetics, 145, 146
  with PTH, 154, 159-160
King, L. S., 40
Klinefelter's syndrome, 97
Knobil, E., 123
Kocher, Emil Theodor, 73
Kosterlitz, Hans, 166-167, 168

Laguesse, G. E., 131
Langerhans, Paul, 130-131
Laron, Zoi, 121
Lerner, A. B., 79-80, 81, 89
Levomorphine, 162
Leydig cells, 101, 107
LH, *see* Luteinizing hormone
LHRH, *see* Luteinizing-hormone-releasing hormone
Li, C. H., 168
Light exposure
  melatonin and, 82-85, 86-87, 89-91
  vitamin D and, 156-157, 158
β-lipotropin, 76, 168-169
Liver, insulin in, 138-140
The Lives of a Cell, 16-17
Loeb, Jacques, 150
Long, J. A., 66, 68, 122-123
Lower, Richard, 37
Luteinizing hormone, (LH), 29, 32, 37, 67-69, 105-114 passim
  LHRH and, 50, 53, 68, 88, 108, 111-112
  pineal gland and, 86, 88-89
Luteinizing-hormone-releasing hormone (LHRH), 44, 47, 50-54, 68, 88, 108, 111-112

MacCallum, W. G., 150
MacLeod, J. J., 129, 133, 135
Magrath, Cornelius, 117
Male pseudohermaphrodites, 96, 104-108
Mandl, Felix, 148-149, 151-152
Marie, Pierre, 60, 61, 66, 68, 117
Martell, Charles, 147-149, 152, 159
Martin, C. J., 9

Massachusetts General Hospital, 159
Matsuo, H., 53-54
M'buti, 121-122
McCann, S. M., 50-51, 52, 54
McCord, C. P., 80
Medulla, adrenal, 24, 25
Meites, J., 54, 56
Melatonin, 79-92
Mellanby, Edward, 155-156
Merck Sharp and Dohme, 46
Merimee, T. J., 121-122
Mering, Joseph von, 131
Messenger ribonucleic acid, (mRNA), 26, 32, 34
Methoxytryptophol, 90
Milk production, mammal, 69-71
Miller, Stanley Lloyd, 3
Minkowski, Oscar, 61, 131
Morphine, 162-163, 164-165, 166, 173
Müllerian regression hormone, 96, 100-108 passim, 112
Murry, George R., 73
Muscles, insulin in, 139-140
Myxedema, 72-73

Naloxone, 164-165, 166, 174
Narcotics, 162-168
  internal, *see* Opioid peptides
National Institutes of Health (NIH), 14, 45, 47
National Pituitary Agency, 123
Nerve damage, with diabetes, 145, 146
Nervous system, 4, 9, 15, 75, 162, 172
  central, 37-40
  sympathetic, 82, 84, 89
Neuroendocrinology, 50
Neurohypophysis, *see* Posterior pituitary
Neuropeptides, 161-176
Neurophysin, 173-174
Neurotransmitters, 4, 14, 15, 168-174 passim
New England Journal of Medicine, 92
Nicolaysen, R., 157
NIH, *see* National Institutes of Health
Nobel Prizes, 44, 133
Non-insulin-dependent diabetes mellitus (NIDDM), 144-145
Normal-variant short stature, 128
N-terminal, 48-49, 50
Nuclear membrane, 29
Nuclear ribonucleic acid (nRNA), 26